6 Tools of the Law of Attraction

Easy tools to use to achieve your dream goal

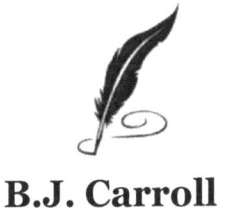

B.J. Carroll

© **Copyright 2021 - All rights reserved.**

The content contained within this book may not be reproduced, duplicated or transmitted without direct written permission from the author or the publisher.

Under no circumstances will any blame or legal responsibility be held against the publisher, or author, for any damages, reparation, or monetary loss due to the information contained within this book, either directly or indirectly.

Legal Notice:

This book is copyright protected. It is only for personal use. You cannot amend, distribute, sell, use, quote or paraphrase any part, or the content within this book, without the consent of the author or publisher.

Disclaimer Notice:

Please note the information contained within this document is for educational and entertainment purposes only. All effort has been executed to present accurate, up to date, reliable, complete information. No warranties of any kind are declared or implied. Readers acknowledge that the author is not engaged in the rendering of legal, financial, medical or professional advice. The content within this book has been derived from various sources. Please consult a licensed professional before attempting any techniques outlined in this book.

By reading this document, the reader agrees that under no circumstances is the author responsible for any losses, direct or indirect, that are incurred as a result of the use of the information contained within this document, including, but not limited to, errors, omissions, or inaccuracies.

Table of Contents

Introduction 1
Chapter 1 5
    Tool One: What is the Law of Attraction? 5
    How do I start the Law of Attraction? 9
Chapter 2 14
    Tool Two: The Importance of Self-Love 14
    The Mind 21
    The Heart 27
    The Body 30
        Acceptance 32
Chapter 3 42
    Tool Three: The Law of Attraction Towards Others 42
Chapter 4 47
    Tool Four: Meditation, Less Stress, and Rest 47
    Meditation 48
        Guided vs. Unguided Meditation 48
        Calming vs. Insight Meditation 49
        Other Forms of Meditation 50
        Ancient Practice Forms 51
        A Few Tips for the Best Meditation 54
    Rest 57
        The Power of the Power Nap 57
Chapter 5 63
    Tool Five: Emotional Freedom Techniques (EFT) and Access Bars 63
        Tapping 64
        Access Bars 67
Chapter 6 69
    Tool Six: Harmony, Right Action, and Moving Your Body 69
    Harmony 69
    The Law of Right Action 73
Chapter 7 76
    The 12 Laws of the Universe 76
    The Law of Divine 77
    Oneness 77
    The Law of Vibration 80
    The Law of Correspondence 84

The Law of Attraction 87
The Law of Right Action... 88
The Law of Perpetual Transmutation of Energy 89
The Law of Cause and Effect 93
The Law of Compensation 96
The Law of Relativity.. 99
The Law of Polarity... 102
The Law of Rhythm 104
The Law of Gender.. 106
Summary of How to Integrate the 12 Universal Laws 108
Conclusion.. **109**
References **110**

Introduction

In 2012, when I had no income and I was living in a foreign country without friends and only two young children, I decided I had time for something new to change my life. It pulled me out of the hole I was stuck in.

I knew what I was doing wasn't working. It wasn't because I wasn't doing *anything* but because I wasn't doing it right. I started searching the internet, enrolling in courses that were supposed to lead me to success.

I even bought the books *The Secret* by Rhonda Bryne and *Money and the Law of Attraction* by Esther and Jerry Hicks.

Even with all the book knowledge I gained, something still wasn't working. I wanted to be a better person and provide for myself and my children.

I wanted to take them on vacation, to dress nicer, lose weight for good, and of course, live in my dream home. Everything described in the books and courses seemed easy to achieve. So, what was I doing wrong?

Today, I found my way. I found how to achieve my goals and make my dreams come true. And I will tell you that it is not, at all, costly. Actually, quite the opposite.

In my life I have had so many past traumas and many false beliefs. They have blocked me from achieving the success I have always dreamed of and desired. But I won, I made it and I am here to tell you that you can too.

So, where to begin? Let's start with what the Law of Attraction is.

The Law of Attraction is a saying most have heard as a buzz phrase. A hairstylist manifests a few good vibes for your new cute hairstyle. Or a friend is wanting to attract a partner.

But do most know the Law of Attraction first appeared in written text at the turn of the 19th century? Helena Petrovna Blavatsky was a spiritual leader in her day. She was thought to be extremely spiritual and often drew most of her teachings from ancient traditions. Madam Blavatsky was an advocate that our reality comes from within ourselves and we are able to move past our own limitations.

The Universe is worked and guided from within outwards – Helena Pertrovna Blavatsky.

As the Law of Attraction took deeper roots, it became something of a phenomenon in the 20th century. Many writers and philosophers began taking their own viewpoints on manifestation to their writings.

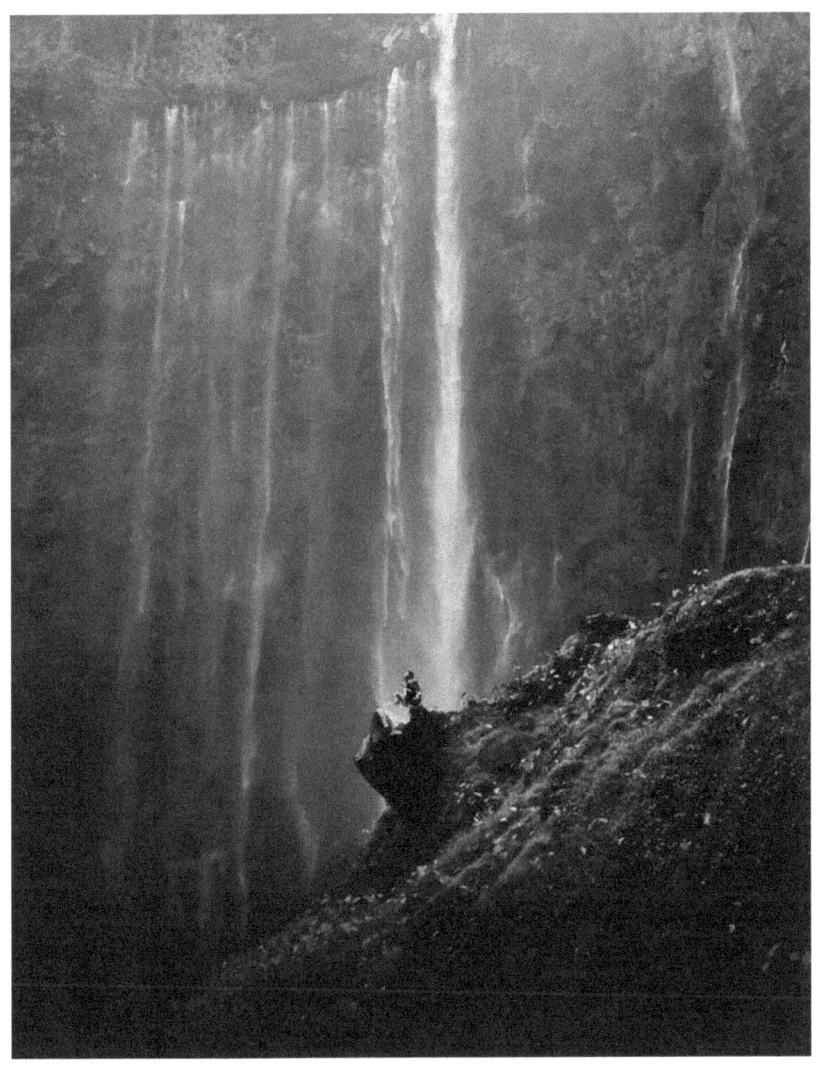

William Walker Atkinson became a prolific practitioner to the Law of Attraction through his belief that the ones who desire to manifest their livelihood should focus on their willpower, strengthening their focus, and manifesting magnetism to bring abundance to their lives. Atkinson drew a majority of his practice from Hinduism which influenced his beliefs about life.

As history and time grew, the 1940's brought a new perspective to modern manifestation. Napoleon Hill chose to take his own route instead of following the teachings of religious scholars like his predecessors. Ralph Waldo Emerson was still an influential writer during Hill's years and Hill developed a more modern attachment to manifestation. He believed negative thoughts will attract negativity into our lives.

The most modern practitioners such as Jerry and Esther Hicks and Louise Hays have developed Hill's practice of positivity to stretch to self-love and compassion.

The Law of Attraction has been around for centuries. Many claim it began from the ancient teachings of Buddha and Hindu teachers. The idea that meditation, balance, and magnetism brings about good things for life isn't a foreign concept. The goal of this guide is to help you understand the root of manifestation and how you can achieve everything you have your heart set on through self-love and good reading.

I can guarantee you there are powerful tools in the world that will change your life, don't be afraid to reach for them!

This book isn't just for the ones who have already dealt with the Law of Attraction before but also for the ones wanting to take the first steps to manifesting their dreams and successes.

Chapter 1

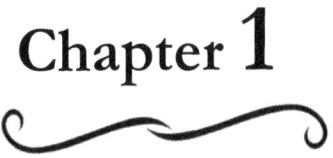

Tool One:
What is the Law of Attraction?

*I*s it a phrase? A saying? Something a funky store puts on T-shirts or a friend comments to you as you leave their house? We've all heard someone say ―sending good vibes to you" but what does it actually *mean* and how does it play a part in your life?

The Law of Attraction, as we've discussed, is not something our culture or generation has created in the past fifteen years. It's lived and thrived across generations, languages, religions, and cultures for centuries. The verbiage may be something we have taken into our modern colloquialisms, but no one should be mistaken that it is something from the current generations.

The Law of Attraction is simply put as positive thoughts bring positive things. In contrast, negative thoughts will bring about negative results to life.

In more complex terms, the Law of Attraction is even related to the Universe. The magnetic, attractive power of the Earth brings about manifestations through everything the Universe touches.

Many may misinterpret the depth of the Law of Attraction, thinking it boils down to wishful thinking. Thoughts like if you concentrate hard enough and never acknowledge negativity, you will get what you are seeking. It is truly much more than that.

It may feel like manifestation hasn't quite worked out for you. Maybe you've been practicing for years and haven't seen any results. A key to remember is if you only focus on what you are wanting, your mind will focus on what you are lacking. Essentially, your brain is a lot smarter than you think. And if you are caught up in the Law of Attraction and only practicing in a way to attract what you don't have, your subconscious will inevitably focus on what you do not have.

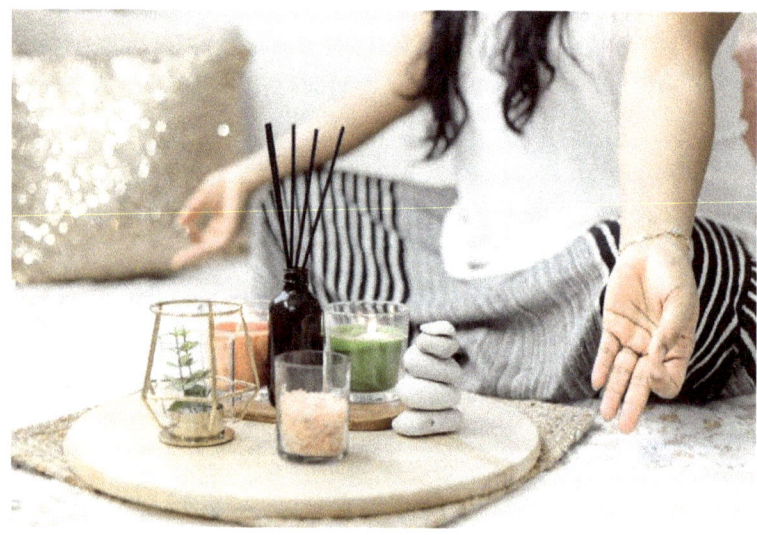

To leave behind the doubtful thoughts of why you don't have something and instead focus on where you want to go brings about true transformation. The conscious mind follows our subconscious thoughts and our body follows our conscious thoughts. It's simple but can be hard to put into practice.

Although, we can't quite control every subconscious thought, if you keep your mind on your goal then your subconscious thoughts will become the one that follows you.

The power of surrender is something profound within the Law of Attraction. It goes something like this; if you are obsessing over a job, your subconscious will only focus on the job you don't have. Surrender your desire. Your mind will give it to the wind and all of the sudden… BOOM! Your dream job is sitting in your hands. Okay, maybe it won't be that immediate but letting go control of your desires releases control over your situation allowing space to come into your life. Space for your life allows you to recognize what you have in front of you instead of what you don't. We will touch on the tool of gratitude later on but it can be an insurmountable gift to release control over situations.

Take a look at your desires. Maybe write them down in front of you and see them physically. How many things are you controlling in your life to make sure you get what you want? It's not a bad thing to have a game-plan, to dream big and go for it, but it might be blocking you from your fullest potential. Once you have them all written out in front of you, connect lines to the reasons you have for wanting to obtain that goal. Your desires or goals in life can look anything from wanting to be married, to owning a home, a career choice, gaining friends, or obtaining a higher self-confidence. Analyze your desires and go through the practice of being honest with yourself. Spend time releasing those desires with open hands.

Have you ever had this situation in your mind before? A person is sitting across from you but they won't look towards you. You decide to go up to them and start up a conversation and nothing comes of it? Your subconscious mind is desiring that person in a way that attracts lack. Instead, turn your mind on what you have in front of you and surrender that person. The magnetism of focusing on what you do have will pull them towards you. If not that person, then someone who will match your vibe better will come along.

The Law of Attraction is practicing self-confidence as well as surrender. Someone who is desperate for love, a job position, a blessed hobby will have a difficult time obtaining these desires.

Why? To first be confident within yourself means to bring confidence in what you are seeking to achieve. Of course, you may be able to land that job or find that person but the odds are it may end in toxicity. You might drive your partner away due to insecurities or lose the job because of lack of initiative due to a lack of confidence. Desperation comes from a lack of self-confidence and sends off inner vibrations that you believe you cannot accomplish what you seek to achieve. Self-love and confidence will be a great thing for you to walk through during your practice of the Law of Attraction.

We'll take a look at how you can begin your journey on the Law of Attraction and all the things that can come into play on this journey!

How do I start the Law of Attraction?

It can feel overwhelming, right? To change your conscious thoughts to then alter your subconscious mind. But there are ways you can jump right in without digging up any of those negative vibes that may block you from your practice!

One of the first steps you can take in the Law of Attraction is to practice gratitude.

Be grateful. Throughout the process we will go over many examples of what things and people you can be grateful for in your life. Below is a process you can do on your own, starting right now.

Take a moment. Now take a breath. Where are you? Be mindful and send gratitude out to where your physical body is at currently. Are your feet on the ground, your heart working, your mind inputting information?

Great! You just took your first steps towards cultivating the Law of Attraction!

Don't be afraid to extend your thoughts of gratitude to the elements; the feel of the air whether hot or cold. The lush sounds of rain falling. The breath that is making its way to your brain.

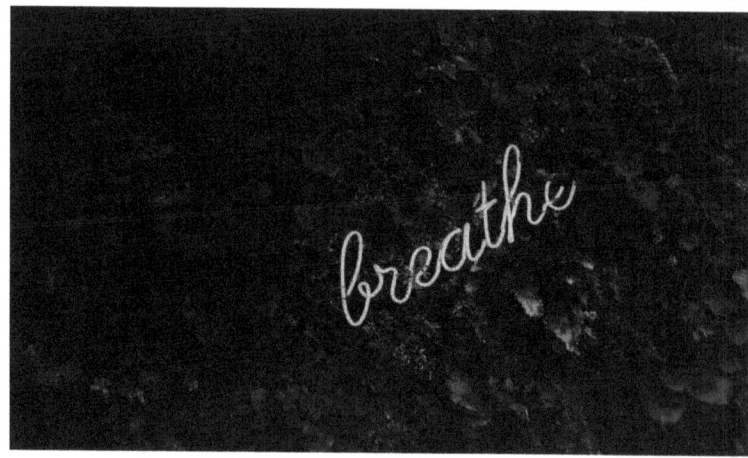

Extend even further to the people you know and love. The ones that have shaped you and helped you back up. Are there people around you? A few random people sitting in the coffee shop you're in? Or in the park walking by you? You may be alone in your home, that's okay. I'm sure there are neighbors that live around you. Send forth gratitude for them and their lives.

What about yourself? The body you hold. The color of your skin, your hair, the color of your nails. The inspiration you hold within. These are all aspects of who you are and they are important.

Gratitude is a great daily practice for anyone who may want to start the journey of manifestation but doesn't quite know where to start. It's easy and goes at your own pace. You may feel lighter even now after your first go at the practice!

Letting go of judgement is a great next step. A lot of time people, circumstances, or even ourselves can create negative magnetic vibrations that only bring similar situations and judgement toward the process can create those negative vibes as well.

Let yourself loosen the grip you have on what you believe you need and what you expect. Allow your mind to accept what makes you happy and the Universe will reverberate those positive vibrations back to you.

If you hate your job and it has created resentment and judgement in your heart, let it go. You may have success and money on your mind but practice the art of surrender and see how the Universe reacts to it. That may be difficult for you. That's okay, it's a hard part of the process. Don't be afraid to do some inner self-realization and acknowledge why you may feel judgement or those negative vibes. Judgement most often comes from a failure we see or feel within ourselves. If this is the case for you, take some time to work through those blocks. To know *you* aren't a failure and to give yourself forgiveness may help you hurdle other forms of judgement in your life. Judgement and resentment are also heavy things to carry along your journey of life anyways. Sit with yourself and gradually learn to let go of those negative vibes.

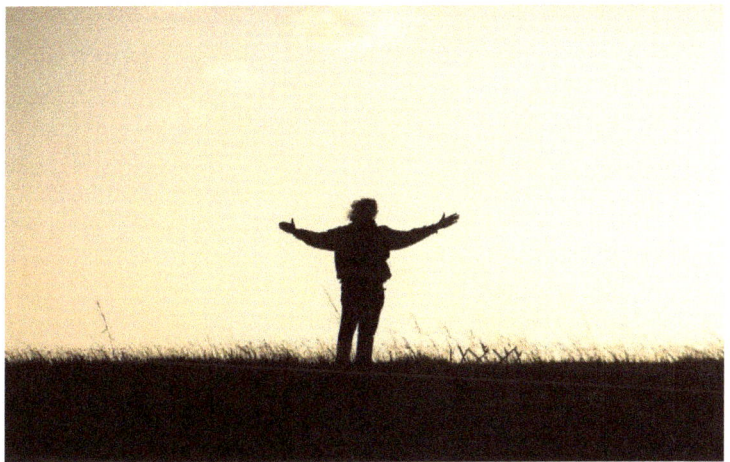

On top of gratitude and releasing judgement, don't sell yourself short.

The Universe is not one to shy away from testing its inhabitants. The Universe may send you a job that is tempting but you know will create judgement and negative thoughts in your mind. Or even a partner that is toxic or berates you down. Don't accept it and don't sell yourself short. To know who you are and what you are worth is invaluable.

Believe in yourself and know you are worth more than what you used to know or what used to be normal. Politely decline to what you know will create negative vibrations and focus on your goal. Something great will come along if you hold true to who you are and how you want to obtain it.

You will change as a person. At a certain time in your life, the Universe may send along exactly what you attract at that specific time. As you grow and change, your mind will become disciplined in the Law of Attraction, morphing you into someone else. As you look back on your journey years from now, you may discover you've been a thousand different forms of yourself. That's okay, that's growth.

Remember to go with the flow and don't hold your hands too tightly around the neck of your desires. Continue to produce gratitude and release judgement from where you once were.

To start your life on the Law of Attraction, truly generate good vibes.

Create gratitude, appreciate what you have, and focus on where you are going. Try not to allow your mind to attach to a desperate want of what you desire your life to look like but allow yourself to be grateful for where and what you have.

You are entirely unique. Your wants, desires, goals, achievements are all things that have developed from how life has shaped you. Be grateful for who and what you have gone through and continue on your journey of life.

Chapter 2

Tool Two:
The Importance of Self-Love

Self-love.

A moment in time where you stop, look in the mirror, and appreciate your body.

A thought that uplifts your value, your worth.

A decision to no longer absorb toxic energy from your boss at work.

The ability to buy yourself that sweet treat.

There are thousands of examples of what self-love can look like. And that's just for one person!

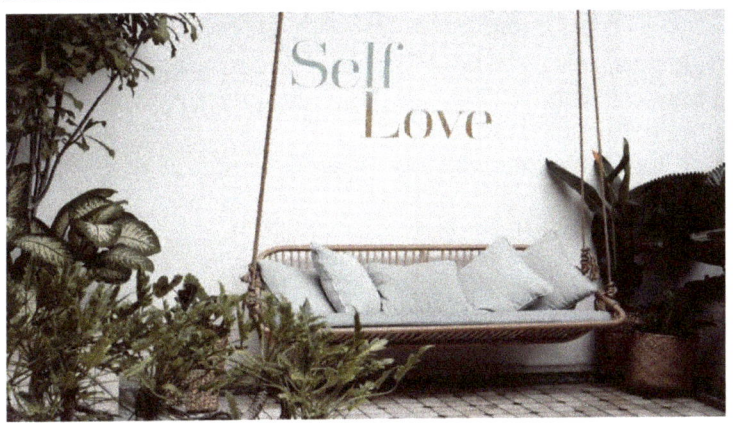

The definition of self-love is entirely personal. You may not relate to a spa day but you may relate to a day laying in a river with cool water lapping over you. The only hard and fast rule to self-love is there are no hard and fast rules. It's simply being who you are and acknowledging what your body and mind needs.

Self-love may be different for everyone but that doesn't mean it is always easy. Many people grew up in toxic homes, created lives that allowed abusive behaviors, or just never learned how to simply *love* themselves. Typically, these are all factors we learned from our guardians as a young child. If you feel anger towards the ones who raised you, it may be beneficial to take some time to go through a few practices to release those vibes. If we are holding onto those emotions of anger, hate, or resentment it can put up blockers preventing us from becoming who we are meant to be. It may even be an act of self-love for you to go through practices that help you release those emotions. Without letting go of what other people have done over us, it will be a long uphill climb to self-love.

Self-love is a journey that is vastly unique. Honestly, it can be a hard path for a lot of people. The best question to ask is what does self-love look and mean to you?

Self-love could look like any of these:

- Putting yourself first
- Silencing self-condemning thoughts
- Trust in yourself
- Belief in yourself
- Healthy and whole boundaries
- Talking with love and gentleness to yourself

A good way to start practicing self-love is to go back to the basics for our bodies and minds. Some practical ideas of loving yourself may look like the list below.

- Stretching everyday
- Making time to groom yourself; Painting your nails, doing your hair, or shaving
- Being creative. Do you enjoy painting? Singing? Dancing? Do that
- Strolls in the park
- Sitting on a bench and admiring nature
- A solo-trip
- Having a pasta and wine night

Reasons why focusing on self-love are extensive. And again, they can also be very individualistic. But a few reasons as to why you should practice self-love include being mindful and knowing yourself. Without self-love and recognizing your needs, it may be a harder journey in becoming altruistic.

Loving yourself also makes time for healthy habits like good rest, exercise, and eating well.

To know yourself means to spend time with yourself. You may be someone who is extremely extroverted. That's great and we completely welcome that. Or you may deal with some deep seated anxiety and feel as though you cannot spend time with yourself. That is a-okay as well. You may feel a rise in anxiety even as you read. But whether we like it or not it is a paramount practice to be able to sit and be with ourselves.

A few ways to practice getting to know yourself are listed below.

- Be still. It may take a lot for you to be still but it's a great practice. Without practicing times where we are quiet and sit with ourselves, how are we going to differentiate who we are from the people we are always with? Again, extroverts are welcome here but know it is valuable to be alone. Introverts may even struggle with being still. Some may like to be alone but are never quiet with themselves. The difference is the work you put in. To be home alone but always on your phone or watching TV doesn't actually mean you are spending time with yourself.

- Acknowledge who you are and not just what you want to be. This is a big one. Many of us take on expectations of who we feel we need to be. Let that go, it's not worth your time. You may have a big corporate job but have always felt inclined to give it all up and live in the desert. Or maybe it's the total opposite. The practice of being still with yourself will help you decide what is you and what is from culture or the influences around you. Many of us have pressures from parents or friends that have guided (or forced) us into a life path that is not our own. Know it will only cause burnout if you continue on that path. Take some time, hang out with yourself, and realize what are your desires and what are other peoples'. If you feel lost on how to find out who you are, take a personality test. There are so many different types that provide insight into who we are as people and what our characteristics are. There's no shame in embracing your zodiac sign or your work style. It's a great tool!

- Discover what you're good at and what you aren't good at. Yes, there is freedom knowing you are not naturally talented at basketball. It doesn't mean you can't play with friends again, but it will give you a release to not put so much pressure on yourself when playing. This step isn't an excuse to quit the things that don't come naturally but hopefully it will give you empowerment to not place as many expectations on yourself. Also, in the same way, realizing what you *are* good at gives you excitement to pursue those things. Maybe you are really good at numbers and you enjoy them but all your friends are painters. You don't need to force yourself to be a painter if you hate it. Embrace what you are good at and release what you feel you should be good at.

- What's your passion? Passion flows right out of discovering what you're good at but there is a difference. Maybe you aren't great at painting but you have a deep passion for it. That's great! Hone into those passions. To know what you are passionate about gives you a great understanding into who you are and allows more ideas to flow into your self-love practice.

- Feedback is key. It may be difficult for some to know where they stop and where others close to them begin. Ask some trusted and reliable friends to speak into who they see and know you to be. This is great for helping you discover who you are and also in building self confidence. Some questions you could ask your trusted acquaintances are, —What do you see some of my strengths are?" Always ask them what they see your weaknesses to be. To successfully do this, you have to be open and trusting of who you are asking. Make sure the people know and love you.

- Know your relationships. A big part of coming to know yourself lives within who you surround yourself with. In the same way, if you don't know yourself then you will never truly know the people around you. Without taking time and insight into yourself as a human being, how will you be able to appreciate those around you? If you're in a relationship but have never given much thought to yourself, then you may be in a relationship you don't truly desire. Again, if you don't know who you are, how will you know who you want to surround yourself with?

It can feel overwhelming to spend time with yourself, analyzing your thoughts, your childhood, fears, and passions but if you break it down all you're really doing is hanging out with yourself! If you're thinking —Why would I want to hangout with myself, no one else wants to hangout with me?", then you are at a point that is paramount to spend time with yourself. You are valuable and you do have things to give to the world. Without spending time with yourself and acknowledging these facts for yourself, you will have a difficult time allowing others to see these traits in you.

A great mantra to keep in mind is to do things because you care about them and not because you feel like you have to get things done. The weight of expectations and obligations we take on from our daily tasks can become tiresome and oftentimes we forget about who we are and what we need. The act of self-love brings us back to what is important and keeps our bodies and minds from burnout.

The importance of self-love is an undeniable asset for the journey of the Law of Attraction. Many may even refer to the practice as the ―Lawof Love". But again, it can be a hard journey in learning how to love yourself.

The Mind

Let's start with the importance of the mind in regards to self-love. Our mental capacity can hold a lot but that doesn't mean it's meant to hold everything within. Emotions are a gateway to the heart and knowing what and how you are feeling is important for your mind to release pressure and expectations. When your mind is holding onto negativity within, it only creates lasting vibrations that will attract more negativity. Releasing negative emotions into the world releases those toxic, negative emotions from inside.

An easy way to start a process of letting go of negative emotions is through talking it out. Ask a friend to sit with you as you process through emotions. Or maybe you are an internal processor and you would rather speak to a piece of paper about your feelings. Even incorporating professional help such as a counselor is always a good way to help your mind release those negative vibrations. Any one of these avenues will help your mind take baggage off of itself and lay it down. Your mind is capable of a lot and that being said, it doesn't need further burdens weighing it down. Relax and allow your mind to take a cleansing breath by releasing those negative thoughts. Later on, in Chapter 4, we will talk about the practice of meditation and how that process can significantly help your mind relax.

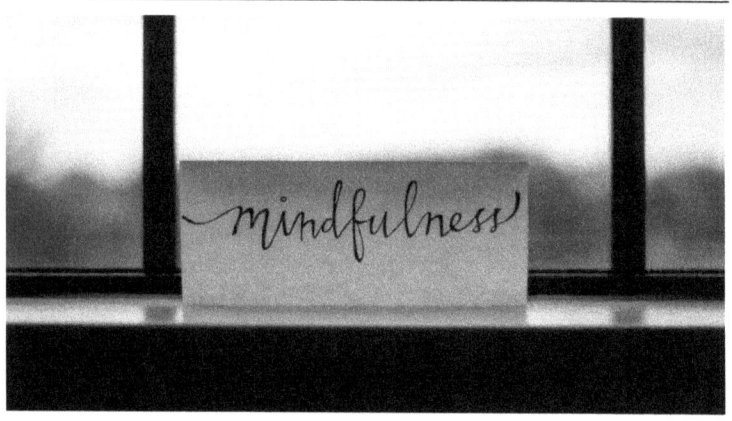

Some people may need more intensive paths for your mind to find self-love. There are therapy sessions individuals can look into if needed.

Eye Movement Desensitization and Reprocessing or EMDR is a form of therapy directly relating to the brain. It was created in the late 20th century and helps people release emotional stressors that typically stem from traumatic events in someone's life. In simple terms, EMDR is performed during a few different sessions. The patient will sit with a therapist and recount the traumatic events affecting the patient either through talking or in the mind. The patient will have different forms of stimulants during this process such as vibrators they hold in their hands or different techniques such as rubbing a leg or arm continually. Then after a short session, the therapist will guide the patient's mind towards something completely unrelated. The back and forth of remembering the traumatic event while also incorporating physical stimulation allows the brain to release stress. This specific type of counselor may be very beneficial to anyone who holds extreme negative self-beliefs, has been through a traumatic event, or even has stressors in life that inhibit you from living freely. More information on EMDR can be found online from the EMDR Institute (see EMDR Institute for more details).

Of course, some may need help with their mental capacity in the form of medicine. Depression, Anxiety, Obsessive Compulsive Disorder (OCD), Attention-Deficit/Hyperactivity Disorder (ADHD), and many other life-prohibiting stressors can cause someone to not be able to give self-love to their minds.

EMDR and medication may be the path you need to take for yourself to find self-love and care for your mind. You may also just need a loving friend who is willing to help you walk through tough thoughts and beliefs you have. Both are perfectly beautiful ways to show your mind that you love and appreciate it.

If you are someone who would rather sit in a quiet coffee shop and release your mind onto a page then I totally relate. There are thousands of prompts, journals, and insights into how you can practice self-love through journaling your heart out.

Let's go through a few journal prompts to get your pen writing through what's on your mind!

Journal Prompts:

1. What feelings do I have about myself as I sit here?

2. What would today look like if I fully honored and loved myself?

3. What do *I* believe self-love looks like? What does it feel like?

4. Are there anxieties I am facing for my day? What are they? Why do I feel anxious?

5. How can I advocate for and promote self-love towards my mind throughout my day today?

6. What things do I need to say no to?

7. Who is inspiring to me? What is it that inspires me?

8. What are 5 things I accept about myself today?

9. Do I receive help from others easily?

10. Where do I block love for myself?

11. How do I compare myself to others and how can I release those comparisons?

12. What am I holding judgments over myself for?

13. What's the best accomplishment I have done for myself?

14. Is there anything I wish others would compliment about me? Am I able to speak about self-love into those areas?

15. What portions of myself do I wish I could change? Can I rewrite them in a way that gives positivity and gratitude towards those specific things?

16. What challenges have I overcome?

6 TOOLS OF THE LAW OF ATTRACTION

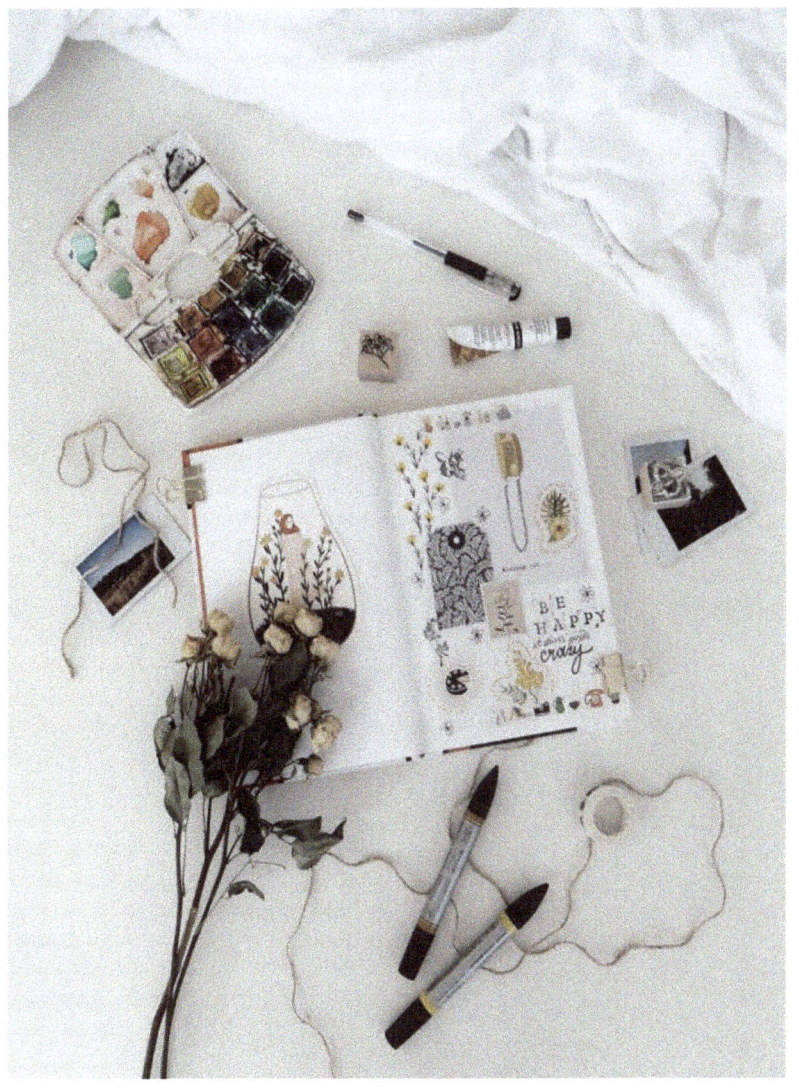

Learning how to process, feel, and release emotions is a great way to start the journey of self-love. Many psychologists claim that bottling up emotions only leads to self-inflicting thoughts. So, learning early on how to walk through what you are feeling will only help in the long-run. Just know you are doing great work and the fact that you are here, taking time to understand yourself and the Law of Attraction is something to honor within yourself.

The Heart

The next easy step in self-love is acknowledging your heart. As you process and release emotions from your mind, keep in mind how you portray these emotions always has a great effect on your self-love. If you do find yourself in a counselor's office, there may be many emotions that come up within your heart. This is very normal and it means you are doing the hard work now to have the best life from this point on.

Many of us are taught that negative emotions are bad emotions. That isn't necessarily true. Anger is an emotion that tells our heart and mind what is going on under the surface level. Anger typically means we feel an injustice towards something or someone. To push those emotions under the surface even further and not acknowledge them only means we will continue to feel them. Or they will come up in different forms that are unfair to the situation or person. If you have a small fight with your boss at work because they took back their word on a promise they made to you and you are angry, work through that. If you don't, that anger might resurface in passive aggressive behavior, only causing more issues at work.

If you feel your heart and emotions are sending your thoughts of worry or fear, acknowledge them. It may be nothing and it could be your brain overriding what the situation is actually portraying. But it also could be something to pay attention to. You know yourself and if you know your instincts are pretty on-point, listen to them. Let's say you could take two different paths home for the night. You could walk through a park and enjoy a quiet stroll or you could walk down the main street. Maybe typically you do take the path through the park but this particular night you feel some worry about that decision. Listen to your instincts and don't wave them away as insignificant. Honor what your heart is speaking to you.

Another way you can check in with your heart is to analyze your intentions. When you sit down to talk with your friend, check in with your heart. Are you able to speak gently with them when they ask questions that may not seem helpful to where you are at? You may be going into a conversation or a setting that you know will not benefit you in the long run. Your intentions may be filled with anger or resentment. Speaking in a cruel or harsh way won't release those negative vibrations from within any more than storing them inside your mind. In the same way, walking into a situation you know is not good for you or your body will not benefit you in the long run. Check in with the intentions in your heart and make decisions accordingly.

To practice self-love through the Law of Attraction, focus on what your heart is saying. Release the positive magnetism you are working at towards the one you are speaking with. The Universe will honor what you are putting out into the world and you will see a release of self-love. You may even be helping the person you're speaking with in the path on the Law of Attraction.

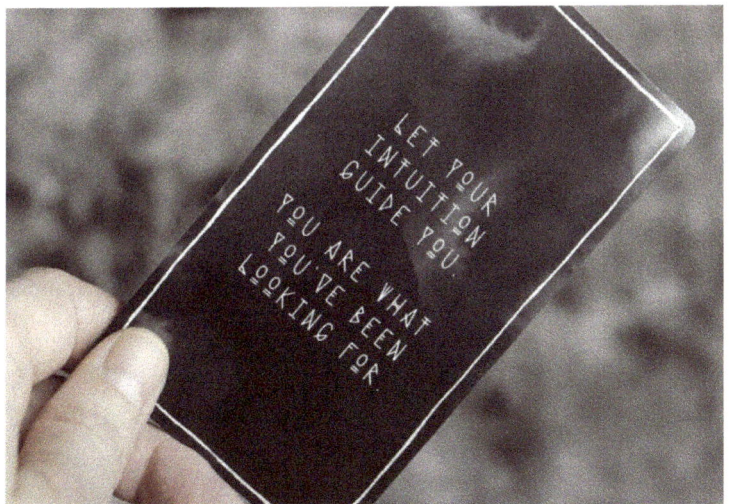

Remember not to accept toxicity into your heart from others as well. If you come to a trusted friend and they sever your trust through their negativity or apathy, take into account how this is absorbed into your heart and take healthy actions. Keep in mind, if someone is speaking harshly or negatively against you then they probably have harsher thoughts towards themselves. What others say to or about you usually doesn't truly reflect on your character. Be strong in who you know you are and you won't be as easily thrown about by what other people think or say. Everyone has magnetism whether they accept it or not, your action is to recognize what they are putting out into the world and react accordingly to where you are in your own journey.

The Body

The body is a great way to practice self-love. It's probably also the easiest way as well. It's the easiest because it doesn't take as much concentration on your inner being. You can move your body and turn your mind off. Some forms of exercise ask for you to be willfully quiet. Yoga is a practice that often allows your mind to wander. Other times running or swimming is a great way to relieve stress and simply move your joints. For others though it may be quite difficult, depending on the person. And I am here to tell you whichever way you are made, is perfectly okay. I believe there is a way for everyone to move their body in a healthy and personalized way!

Of course moving your body is one way to practice self-love. This does not mean you have to be athletic but it is proven that your body needs and craves exercise.

You might hate cardio, that is perfectly fine! Maybe choose a light circuit of yoga. You may hate stretching, all good here, how about boxing? Finding the best way for you and your body to move will be helpful in your journey of self-love. Self-love, especially bodily, is not a linear path. One month you could choose running and the next you are lifting weights. Give yourself time and freedom to flow with what your body is craving. Don't be afraid to go outside your comfort zone by moving your body. Trying water aerobics may be your new hobby, but you'll never know if you don't give it a try.

You may also come to find that moving your body can help you align your mind and heart as well. Nature is a perfect example. Being in nature puts us in a natural element away from the hustle and bustle of everyday life. Taking a hike will get your blood pumping, cleanse your lungs, give space to your mind, and even help you create enough stillness to acknowledge your heart. You may not be a huge hiker. Even going on a mile walk and choosing to walk through the path in your local arboretum can be just as refreshing as the Rocky Mountains.

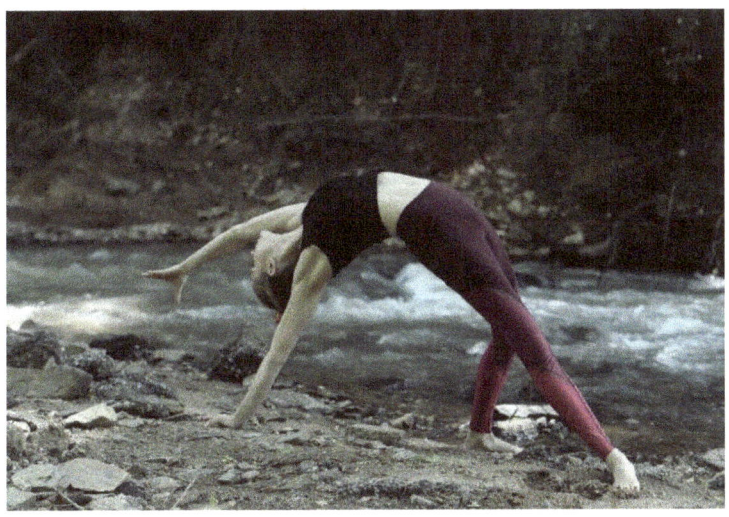

Self-love for the body doesn't just mean being active. Another way you can practice self-love towards your body can be something called mirror work.

I've heard of people taking out all the mirrors in their home because it causes such a negative effect on their well-being. It doesn't have to be this way. Mirror work is simple but also very difficult, especially if you struggle with self-image. But I encourage you that it can be very impactful. To start mirror work all you do is look at the mirror and tell yourself a loving sentence. Start with —love you." It may feel very silly but it's probably something you need to hear. Or you can change it up to be something entirely different. To speak confidence, love, and importance to yourself is essential. Try and do this once a day and from there, work your way up to every time you look in a mirror.

To know when you need to practice self-love to your body takes introspection of your heart and mind. To get started here is a list of questions to consider when deciding how to take action in loving your body.

1. Are you overwhelmed or underwhelmed in life?

2. When you sit alone, what does your body crave? Silence and stillness or energy and activity? Keep in mind, one is not better than the other.

3. If your body is craving stillness, consider lighting a few candles, turning off your lights, and drawing a hot bath. Give your body space to be.

4. If you feel yourself craving energy, maybe go for a walk in your favorite park, ask a close friend to get a drink, or even get a group together to play some card games.

Bodily self-love looks different for everyone. And that is the beauty of the practice. Whatever brings you peace and joy, do that with open hands. The best practice for your body will probably change as you evolve and grow. Don't hold your practice too firmly but allow flexibility for your body (pun intended)!

Acceptance

Self-love is acceptance. Acceptance of mind, heart, and body. What you accept to live with shapes who you are. To accept what the Universe has given you is to accept the magnetism you were empowered to possess. Only you can give off that specific magnetism. Embrace it.

To accept that you have a difficult time with self-criticizing thoughts is the first step to help make change within yourself. The Universe may be sending you some hard things at the moment; it's okay to feel the full force of those vibrations and also come to terms with it.

To accept your body takes people years to conquer, maybe even a lifetime. When you were a child, the voices you heard from people surrounding you may have been extremely negative or nonexistent. Now it is your turn to change the pattern. Learn how to acknowledge your body. The curves, the metabolism, the color, and texture are all yours and no one else's. No one can take them from you and no one can speak power over them except the people you allow to have a voice in that area. Many people have struggled with eating disorders, body dysmorphia, and many other self-inflicting thoughts that cause you to degrade the vessel you were given. To accept the body you were given is powerful and can, quite frankly, change your world. Our bodies hold so much for us. Within them they hold our loves, passions, ideas, heart, brain, and memories.

But I won't sit here and tell you that body positivity will be something you hold within yourself every minute of every day. That is not realistic. And if you hold yourself to a standard of body positivity in every moment, the reality is you are setting yourself up for failure. That expectation is a very high one and it may feel more like a heavy weight to carry rather than freedom. But in the moment you don't feel ecstatic about your body, give yourself grace and space to sit in those emotions. Come back to a mindfulness of what your body holds and accept those emotions of negativity. It will be better for your mental and heart health to accept even the negative moments rather than act like they do not exist.

Another way to bring acceptance to your body is by not allowing those negative voices from the outside in. What I mean by this is if you have friends or family members who say passive comments about your looks and outer appearance, do the healthy thing and do not allow them to speak into that part of your life. We've all heard comments whether it be directed at us or someone else. They usually sound something like, "Oh, you're getting another serving?" or "Are you sure you want to wear those pants?". Passive aggressive comments like these are hard to not accept into your mind and space but not allowing those words to have any authority in your life will help you with your own journey of body positivity.

Body acceptance doesn't just look like body positivity, it can also look like accepting the limits of your body and honoring them. You could have been a professional athlete at one point but now you're a bit older and your body doesn't bend in the same way. Or maybe you won track meets in high school but now you find the faster you run the worse your body feels. Honor that and listen to your body. Our bodies grow as they need and when you find your body is in worse shape than it was before you did that workout, maybe take a step back. A bit of soreness isn't a bad thing, that usually means our muscles are becoming stronger but if you find your body sore, injured, or unable to move because you are trying to push the same limits you did at 17, maybe it is time to reevaluate. Acceptance of the body means different things for a lot of different people. Spend some time with yourself today really listening to the needs of your body and accept it for what it is.

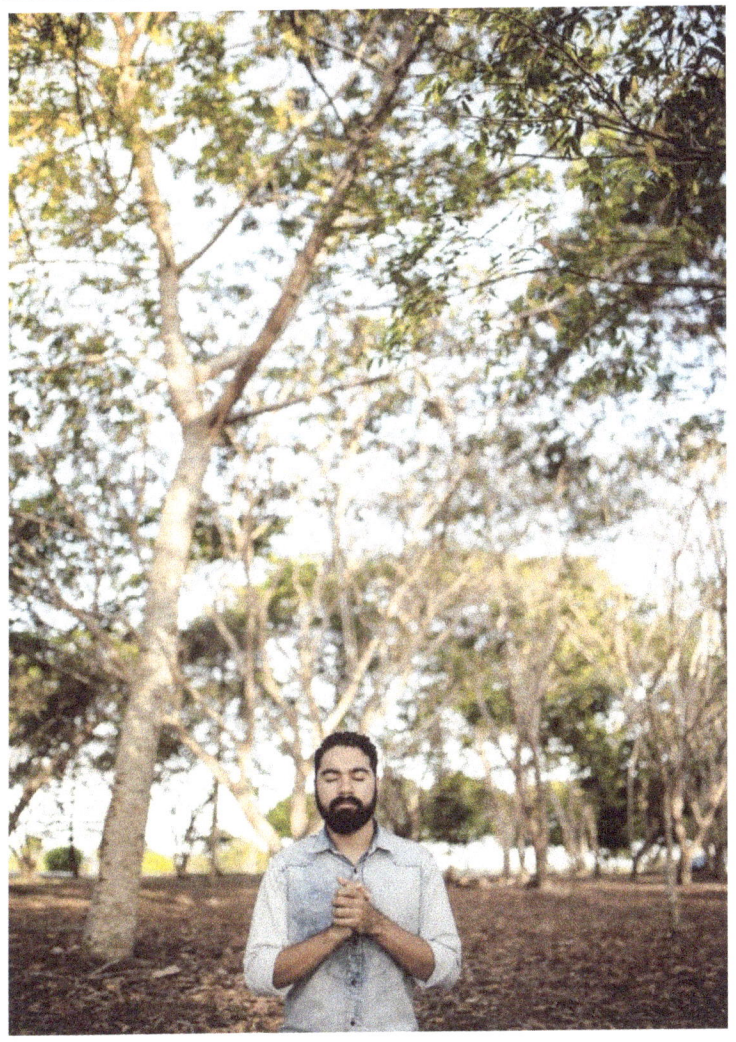

Body neutrality is another concept that goes far with acceptance of the body. This idea says there is no good or bad relating to your body but only what is. Our culture holds a perverted view of what body positivity is. The conversation is changing to something a little more healthy but it still revolves around the idea that every body shape is beautiful except our own. Another way of saying this is you see a person walking down the street and you think to yourself, ‒They are really rocking their skin", and then you look at yourself and think, ‒I should've worn something a little less tight." You are, either consciously or subconsciously, comparing your body to theirs even if you just reimbursed body positivity for that specific person. So, body neutrality is looking at yourself and saying, ‒This is what I have and I know I need to honor and love it." Without judgment or a higher standard for yourself than others, body neutrality is an important conversation to have with yourself.

To accept your body, it takes some inner work with your heart and mind. But the work of accepting your heart and mind is just as important as the body.

I knew a girl once who was diagnosed with a certain neurodiversity. She hated herself. For years and years she thought she was unworthy, unloveable, and odd. When I would sit down to chat with her, the life stories she retold were covered in shame and embarrassment as a young kid and teenager of what life gave her. But as she grew older she found people, or people found her, who embraced all that she was. It took years for her to come to a place of acceptance of the mind she was given but now she often looks back and laughs at how shallow her thinking used to be of herself. She came into an acceptance of her mind and blossomed into an open and joyful person. Maybe your story doesn't involve a neurodiverse mind, or maybe it does, but the process of learning acceptance of our mind can be quite the journey.

A great practice to start, if you feel you could work on accepting your mind, is repeating truths to yourself daily. Maybe that looks like my friend who had people surrounding her telling her the truth they see within her. Or maybe it's you, in your room, doing the hard work and repeating that you are loveable and worthy of space. Either way that fits who you are is beneficial.

Something that could help this process is blessing other people with truths you see within them. I am an advocate for knowing, accepting, and loving yourself first before enacting what you've learned to the world. But in some cases, it can be quite helpful to put some practice into speaking truths out into the open. Maybe you could start with the barista you see on your way to work. Let them know they hold space that is worthy and they are exactly where they need to be. Finding those little moments to send some self-love out to others can help you see for yourself that you are just as loved.

The art of letting go may be a game-changer for you. How many times a day do you revisit the conversation you had with a coworker, thinking of all the better responses you could have given? Or when you got upset at your Uber driver for being late or taking a wrong turn? Many people struggle with self-inflicting thoughts that have to do with situations they feel they could have handled better. The best thing you can do when you are faced with those endless conversations with yourself is to let it go. That may seem like a hard concept to practice and you may be saying to yourself that you have tried that before and you can't seem to release it. If that is the case, it may be good for you to enter into a time of meditation and spend some space asking yourself questions.

If you do find that it's hard to let go of conversations or situations you could have handled better, ask yourself these questions and spend some time meditating over them:

- Do I find it hard to let go of badly handled situations because I have a hard time forgiving myself?

- Do I need to allow my mind to forgive myself for things I could have controlled better?

- Do I have a hard time with self-forgiveness because I have a hard time accepting that I am not perfect?

- Am I perfect? If not, is that okay?

The reason most have a hard time letting those situations go is because they have a hard time either realizing they need to forgive themselves or they have a hard time realizing they are allowed to forgive themselves. It comes down to pridefulness, essentially. The best fact is choosing to give yourself forgiveness does not mean you're weak. It does not mean what happened to you or what you did to someone else is acceptable and it doesn't mean you accept toxic behavior. Forgiveness does mean you are willing to accept what happened and let it go. Once you walk through forgiving yourself, there is no longer any reason to self-inflict. But, forgiveness of yourself can be a lifelong journey.

So, let's go back to the idea of meditating. To start out with asking yourself the above questions is a great way to have a healthier and more understanding sense of your inner self. It's probably a good idea to know why you hold onto those situations for so long and how to move forward in it. Once you realize if you have more tendencies to not feel like you need forgiveness or feel like you don't deserve forgiveness will help you take the next steps as well. Being willing and humbled in this process is key to a healthier acceptance of your mind.

When you take the steps to forgive yourself, several things need to happen.

- Accept responsibility for the situation that happened. If you yelled at your cab driver, accept it. Take responsibility for how you acted, don't shy away from it or act as if how you acted was justified.

- Give your heart and space time to grieve what happened. This doesn't have to mean sobbing on the floor, or maybe it does for you, but it does mean allowing yourself to feel sad, remorse, or guilt for what happened.

- Release the weight of what you did by acknowledging it has happened, you've taken responsibility for it, and you've grieved what you have done.

The act of self-forgiveness is a powerful act but, as stated before, a difficult one. It may help you if you know the correct way to apologize to someone else as well. You can take the steps of apologizing to another person and apply it to yourself.

Apologizing to someone else requires a few things. Most people are taught as kids that if you do something wrong to someone, you say sorry and hug it out. But we all know as little kids the act was meaningless to us and we just did it so we could keep playing outside. So what are the steps to apologizing? It goes something like this:

I'm sorry for doing (state action), I know it made you feel like (state how the person has expressed it made them feel; neglected, unloved, hurt). I am sorry, will you forgive me? Is there anything I can do next time to improve how I handle the situation?

The proper apology heals the person it is addressed to and also takes responsibility for what you did. You can practice the same apology with yourself and release forgiveness to yourself.

Practicing these steps may help you release the weight of shame and guilt you feel over handling situations poorly.

You may not have handled a situation poorly but because you have such high expectations for yourself, it can feel like you have done something wrong. If that is the case, spend some time evaluating that for yourself. Where does it stem from? How are you enabling those emotions? Are the people around you supporting you or reimbursing the negative feelings you already feel?

Have you ever heard the phrase that the heart is 18 inches from the brain? The meaning behind this is it takes a while for things to go from the head to the heart. All these things we have talked about takes time and effort. Accepting that your heart may be slower to accept new truths and habits than your brain is okay.

If you've been practicing self-care for years but are still struggling to believe you deserve self-care, recognize that. And know that your heart may still need a bit more time to fully understand that for itself.

Be aware that to know something is different then to accept something as true to yourself. The key to acceptance of the heart is compassion for yourself.

The habits, decisions, and paths you are choosing to stop in its tracks by accepting and loving yourself is a hard mission. They are things that have been embedded within you as a child.

Give yourself extra time and compassion for your heart to catch up to your head in acceptance.

Of course all of this is easier written than enacted but taking small, mindful steps each day towards acceptance of the mind, heart, and body is a great way to start your path into the Law of Attraction through self-love.

Chapter 3

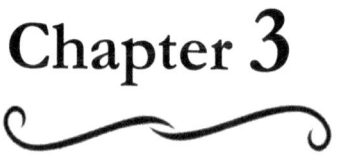

Tool Three:
The Law of Attraction Towards Others

The Law of Attraction is a work in progress, something you will continue to learn and grow in every day. Alongside the inner work that needs to be done to flourish, the outer work comes along with it. One is an input and one is an output.

There are a few different avenues the Law of Attraction flows into regarding manifestation towards others. You can manifest magnetism to attract someone, manifest the right vibrations to bring the job you're desiring towards yourself, or even coach someone else through the Law of Attraction through your actions towards them.

Let's start with the Law of Attraction and the practice of vibrations towards someone else. Most of us have an ideal partner in mind. Someone tall and quirky with brown hair and a really creative job you've always admired. Or the person who values success and material goods who is kind, helpful, and there for you. It's not a bad thing to want what you want but it can get in your own way when you are wanting to bring someone towards you.

The energy your body gives off when desiring something or someone can be very strong. And again, whether others know it or not, they can feel these energies.

The key to understanding how to attract someone towards yourself is by finding a person who is practicing the same amount of vibrations you are.

What this means is the other person has to be seeking to be vibrationally aligned in the Universe in the same way you are. If a person isn't seeking that, they will be falling into toxicity, negative vibrations, or simply won't know how to react to your energy.

So, how do you know if a person is vibrationally aligned with you? Continue doing what you've been doing. And they will continue what they have been doing, and eventually the Universe will pull you together. This doesn't mean do nothing. No, you do have to take action. Say you're at a bar and the atmosphere is exactly what you need, strike up a conversation with the person you are interested in. Hear and see their vibrations and if they are aligned, they will hear and see yours.

If you have studied the Law of Attraction before, you've probably read these three words: Ask, Believe, Receive. But there may actually be a fourth word that needs to be included... Act.

If you are wanting to attract a love into your life, continue being grateful for what you currently have and take steps to work towards self-love but don't think the Universe will simply place someone at your door. The Universe might and if so, I would love to hear about it! But if not, don't forget the fourth important word: Act. Take action for what the Universe puts in front of you with an open hand. If something comes along and you think this is what you have been asking for but it doesn't work out, let it go. If anything, it will teach you how to continue in gratitude for what you have currently.

You may not be asking for someone specific in your life but you may be asking for that perfect job or success to be able to achieve your dreams or provide for your family.

To start the journey down the path of what you desire within a career it's best to start with a vision board. I'm sure you've heard of this before and maybe as you read you're feeling defeated because you're looking at your fourth vision board this month!

Don't feel discouraged. Let's take a closer look at how you can start (or restart) a vision board.

- Keep in your mind's eye the career you are hoping to achieve. What is it? Get specific.

- Set realistic goals for yourself. If you want to be a fashion designer, you probably shouldn't have your first step be applying at Gucci. Make a list of small steps leading towards what you are wanting to achieve.

- Identify your abundance blocks. Abundance blocks are subconscious thoughts you hold that put roadblocks in your way. Identifying these blocks and being honest with yourself is a mighty step.

- Learning how to utilize your tools correctly is essential.

- Take action accordingly.

We'll go through each point of your vision board together so you have an idea of what it could look like.

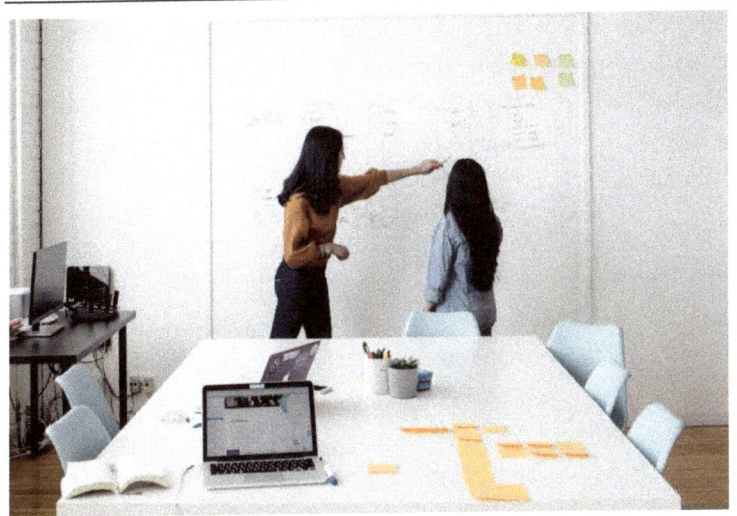

What career are you heading towards? A general idea such as ‚writing' can be very vague to start out with. It may be hard to identify the exact path you want to take but do some research and self-inspecting and try to be as specific as you can be.

Now that you have identified the specific career you are wanting to achieve, set goals. Let's say you have landed on ‚content writer'. What goals could you set? How about starting a journal you write in every day to test your abilities and stretch your skills. Maybe go to some creative writing readings to hear the ebb and flow of sentences. Set a goal to read a certain amount of books about writing by a certain date. These are small steps but probably don't feel as overwhelming as walking into your favorite authors' publishing firm and handing in your resume. Unless, of course, you're ready for that step!

Abundance blocks can be all over your brain. And they could have started from a very young age. A family member may have told you because English is your second language, you'll never be a writer. A bad grade in school discouraged you from continuing in that specific class. These are all abundance blocks. They literally block the abundance from within you to succeed in your achievements and goals. Analyzing your subconscious is difficult but it may be what you need.

When we allow abundance blocks to continue in our lives they encourage insecurities, negative thoughts, and sometimes hopelessness. Meditation is a great way to sit with your own mind to acknowledge these blocks. When you do sit with yourself, be kind to your mind. Remember what you have learned through self-love and don't aggressively push away these blocks. Accept them, welcome them, and let them go into the Universe as best as you can. We all have abundance blocks but when you release the power they have over your mind, you will start seeing real change.

Everyone has tools they were given. Tools of communication, love, desire, determination. Acceptance is key. Walk into what you were given, manifest the power to control your tools and skills and focus them to what you are desiring to achieve.

Chapter 4

Tool Four:
Meditation, Less Stress, and Rest

*I*t's common knowledge that lowering stressors and focusing on your rest is a huge help to any mental block or unresolved emotions. Rest is found to improve your overall health. Sleeping stores the day's knowledge and stresses in your brain to allow a fresh start to the next day. But sleep isn't the only way to obtain rest. Some people are only able to sleep four to five hours a night. Others have such busy lives and jobs, there simply isn't enough time to stay in bed for eight to nine hours.

The good news is there are other ways to rest your mind and body. One of the most taught and ancient practices is meditation.

Meditation

Meditation is the practice of bringing your mind and body to stillness. To bring both to a point of peace and tranquility has kept people studying the practice for a lifetime.

I'll walk you through a few stages of mediation and some practices for each to get you started. The key to meditation is taking the time to discover which practice suits you best. There is no right or wrong form of bringing stillness into your inner being.

Guided vs. Unguided Meditation

The first step in meditation is asking yourself if you prefer guided or unguided practices. This means do you enjoy someone with you as you breathe in and out, speaking to you about what to allow to flow into your time of stillness or not. If your answer is a yes, then I would suggest looking into guided meditation times. This can look vastly different in-and-of itself. You could seek out a teacher in your local area, have a friend sit with you and prompt you to breathe and clear your mind, or even download an app. There are hundreds of creative ways you could begin your guided meditation journey. Guided meditation is a great first step to open your eyes and heart on how to begin your stillness and how to incorporate this time in your daily life.

Unguided meditation is simply you are alone in your practice. Instead of having a guide or teacher walk you through the process, it is just you. Normally, this would look like choosing a peaceful place where you know you won't be interrupted. Next, focus on your body and breathing.

Acknowledging the thoughts that float into your mind and release them. Keep coming back to your breathing and body throughout the practice and take into account the space your mind is taking up.

Of course you can practice a variation of the two. That is the magic of meditation. There truly isn't a form to it. If one day you feel you would enjoy someone walking you through the process, press play on your app. If you feel you need complete space and silence, listen to your body and be still.

Calming vs. Insight Meditation

Meditation can either be a time of peace and calming waves of silence or a time to reflect on the world and yourself in it.

Calming meditation tends to focus more on cultivating a quieter inner being. This practice helps with concentration and peace of mind. This practice usually involves focusing on a certain attribute or physical presence. You can choose your body, taking into account the stress you hold in your shoulders. A clenched jaw or maybe a furrowed brow. Release the pressure and focus on quieting your body. Or focus on your breath. In and out, in and out. Potentially take a full lungs-worth of breath and let it out slowly. Calming meditation is all about releasing a calming balm of quiet energy over your body and mind.

Insight meditation is often focused on an intention you want to cultivate within your inner being. Whether it be compassion, kindness, love, or even mindfulness this is a great place to start. It is similar to calming meditation in that you focus on your breath but while breathing, take note of what thoughts come to mind. Flow with your mind, breathing in compassion and breathing out apathy.

Other Forms of Meditation

A practice called **Noting** is important for everyone to take into their routine at some point or another. Sit in a quiet space and begin taking note of what thoughts or actions drift into your mind. Our world is so fast and it can be hard to know what your subconscious is thinking on a daily basis. Noting is a perfect way to see what emotions you may be ignoring or inner thoughts you need to confront.

Visualization is when you bring a picture to the forefront of your mind. Many therapists have their patients practice this when walking through hard traumas. Let's start with an easy example. If you really enjoy the beach, bring your favorite beach to the forefront of your mind. Focus on your senses. The warm heat basking your skin with Vitamin D. The waves that are a consistent noise and continue to crash back to the shore. The wind on your skin, wiping away moisture. The smell of salt and sweet food. Conjure your peaceful place in your mind and spend some time bringing your mind back to this place when it wanders.

If you are having difficulty letting go of negative emotions towards someone, maybe you should give the practice of **Loving Kindness** a try. Imagine the person, or it may be an event, in your mind and release good intentions towards them. This practice will help you release negative emotions or thoughts and allow you to get past the mountain of resentment. I advise you to practice this in the care of a professional, especially if you are bringing forth extremely painful memories or traumas.

Reflection, in a similar way to noting, brings you to an action stance towards meditation. Before going into your practice, write down or have in your mind a question you would like to walk through. Maybe it's —"What are you most grateful for?" Focus on your emotions, not your intellectual thoughts during this practice. Asking in the third person will help you disassociate your thoughts from feelings.

Ancient Practice Forms

There are truly thousands of forms of meditation and it depends on the person, place, and timing of practice which one you will choose. But below I have put a list of a few more that may come in handy for your practice.

- Zen Meditation: Sit in an upright and straight position. Typically, cross your legs and have your shoulders back. Focus on breathing from your stomach and allow your mind to flow. Aim to bring about attentiveness and presence.

- Mantra Meditation: Instead of focusing on a person or event, like the Loving Kindness practice, bring to mind a word or phrase. Different from focusing on your breath, focus on this mantra. The small vibrations of repeating the mantra out loud will stimulate positive changes within you.

- Transcendental Meditation: This meditation style typically involves a trained professional to walk you through the process. This is usually a twice a day practice. You will sit with your eyes closed for 20 minutes as your professional teacher guides you through the process.

- Yoga Meditation: Yoga comes in many styles and fashions but one that focuses on meditation is called Kundalini. Kundalini is directed at encouraging the nervous system to strengthen. This practice helps us to be able to take on the everyday pressure of life and it's stresses.

- Vipassana Meditation: Non-self, unsatisfactory, sufferings, aloneness; these are all human attributes that Vipassana targets. To sit and intently focus on the human experience as we exist forces us to take into mind what we think and believe in each of these aspects. Vipassana pushes one to reach transformation.

- Chakra meditation is a famous practice. There are a lot of adaptations in movies, books, and in the world. But opening up your chakras and aligning them is a great meditation practice. Your body's core holds your chakras and when these are not aligned, open, and fluid, your body becomes sick mentally and physically.

- To help bring healing energies into your body and send out healing energies to others, try using the Qigong meditation. This Chinese ancient practice opens up energy pathways called ‚meridians' creating open and fluid energy that flows in and out of the body.

- Sound Bath meditation uses gongs, symbols, or vibrating instruments to help center the mind and bring the body to the present while meditating. The energy through the vibrations strengthens the focus of the mind.

Rest is an essential part of the process of meditation. Many of these practices will bring rest into your daily life naturally so it's a good idea to aim to sit in stillness frequently.

The old saying is if you can't find time to meditate for 10 minutes, then you need 20. Essentially, this means if you are too busy for 10 minutes of stillness then you probably need it more than you know.

The average person spends most of their day in thoughts that either lead to more stress or come to dead ends. This looks a lot like reviewing the way you could have pitched your idea better to your boss. That thing you did when you were 16 that you are worried will still affect your life. All these thoughts take a huge mental toll on the stillness of your mind which directly relates to the quality and health of your life.

The best time to meditate is in the morning. You just woke up from sleep, your day is beginning and it's going to be full of rushing from one side of the to the other, picking up kids, getting groceries, catching up with friends. Why not take the quietness of the morning to prioritize meditating. It brings fresh awareness to your body. Focusing on how much your body can accomplish today, recognizing that, and respecting your body. Leaning into your mind, doing a scan of your feelings and emotions. Take into account how much energy you feel and what you can do to honor your mind throughout the day. The morning is typically found to have the least amount of distractions. But of course, if the morning isn't the ideal time, find a time that is for you. Maybe during your lunch or your walk through the park on your way home. Any time spent meditating will surely improve your focus, health, and well-being for the day.

When you do head into your time of stillness there are a few tips that can help you focus on your process. Try leaving your phone in a different room. We all know the random pings can bring us out of whatever we were thinking or focusing on. But sometimes silencing our phones isn't enough, I encourage you to put it in a different room than you are in. Out of sight, out of mind.

Find a room that isn't cluttered with things to do. Do you have a room that's without a TV or your computer? Sit in front of a window, allowing the sun to shine through the windows on you and begin to breathe deeply to let your mind rest. The best thing you can do is be consistent in your practice. Incorporating it every day will make it a part of your daily routine. Remember meditation is completely your own, so don't be afraid to adapt and change what needs to be tweaked when something isn't working.

A Few Tips for the Best Meditation

1. Early bird gets the best stillness. You don't have to be up at the crack of dawn, or even a morning person, but one of the best things you can do is incorporate your practice into your morning routine. There are a few benefits to sunrise meditation. You're able to think clearly and give your mind space before the day begins. Then you will be able to check it off your to-do list for the rest of the day. Meditation should not become a burden, then it might become counteractive, but you will be able to focus stillness into the rest of your day knowing you started out with something beneficial.

2. 9 a.m. next to the couch. Okay, maybe 10:30 a.m.? Whatever time works best for you, even if that's not the morning, try to aim to have your meditation in the same place and at the same time. To have your body into the routine of sitting everyday at the same time is great for nurturing your body into a new habit.

3. Be creative. Everyday you wont be able to sit down at the same time and in the same place for a 10 minute meditation session. So when those days do arise, be flexible with yourself. The practice of meditation can be done anywhere so where you go, it comes with you. If you have a long ride home, embrace the stillness and

walk yourself through a time of meditation. Or if you feel the need to go on a walk by yourself, what a great opportunity to focus on stillness!

4. Lay on your back, hang your head off your bed. The stereotypical position of criss-cross-applesauce isn't needed here. Most find this position uncomfortable especially if you are sitting on the ground. So sprawl those legs out, lay with your head on a pillow. This practice is for you so don't force your body into an uncomfortable position when it isn't necessary.

Once you're done meditating, take a few moments to check in with yourself. Oftentimes a meditation session can bring up some unwanted emotions or intrusive thoughts. Other times, you could feel completely free and go on with your day. But if you do feel yourself edging into those territories, honor that and take a few moments to observe. Are you feeling certain emotions? Why? What caused these anxieties or feelings? Honor what you feel and it may be something to take note of the next time you practice.

Meditation is not always the easiest thing to remember or incorporate. If you find yourself skipping days, take some notes. Write down your excuses and the next day they won't hold so much power over your mental and bodily status.

Having a companion to join you in your time of meditating is great. It not only bonds you closer to a friend but keeps you accountable in your own practice. Isn't it fun to chat with someone about similar experiences you have? We all love doing it. So why not bring a friend along the way as you discover the art of stillness.

Lastly, don't be too harsh with yourself or your practices. Judgement is something that needs to fly away with every other bad energy your body holds. There truly is no right or wrong, no good or bad form of meditation. Take pride that you are taking the right steps for the best physical and mental health you can have in this life. Also, let your judgments of your friends' practices fly out the door of your heart as well. If this is something you have found yourself thinking, maybe it's time you sit with those emotions in your practice and allow gratitude to come in and judgment out.

Rest

On top of meditation, which itself is a form of rest, there are many different approaches to resting your body that can benefit your well-being and help stimulate the Law of Attraction in your life.

The Power of the Power Nap

What a beautiful phrase, right? Who doesn't want to hear that taking a short nap once a day can reenergize you and prepare you for the rest of your day! There are a lot of questions surrounding the so-called 'power nap', like how many minutes counts as a power nap?

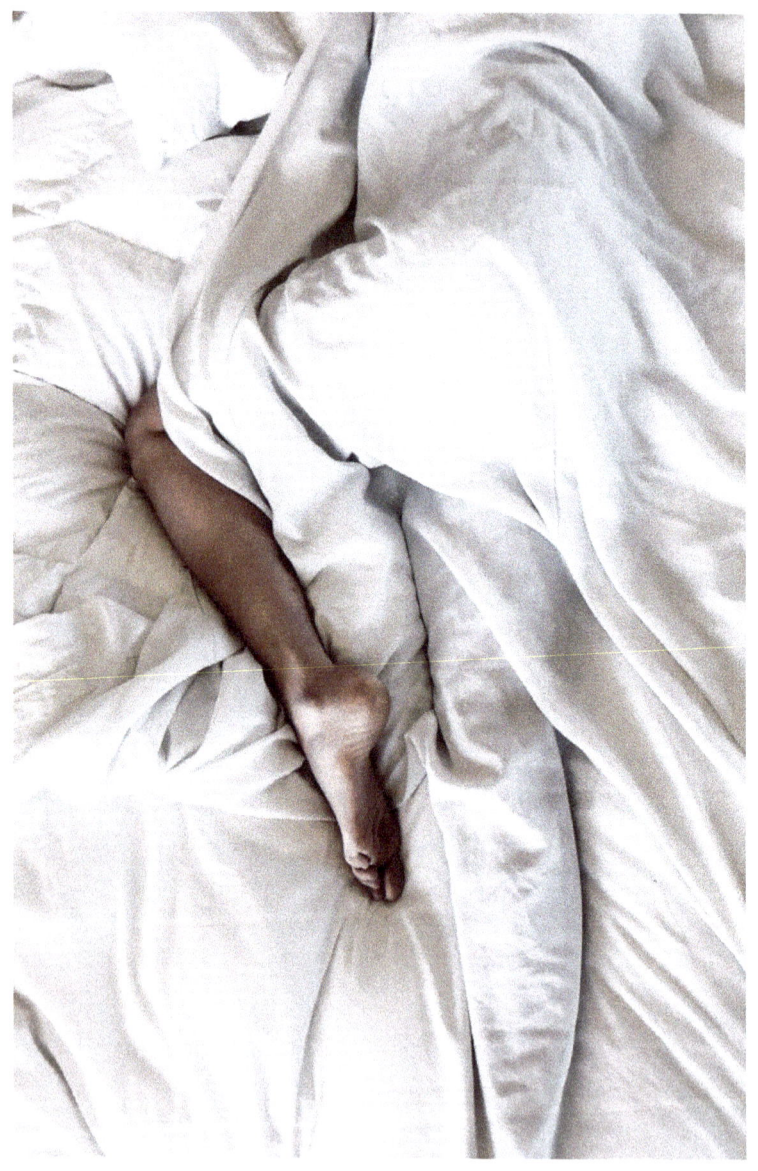

I would guess many would like to hear that an hour long nap is the best case scenario for your day. A nice warm blanket, maybe some black out curtains but to much dismay, the long naps aren't the best for your body. Power naps can help if you tend to go to bed later than you might want to admit or if you usually stay up late working. But these types of naps usually work best when someone has a regimented sleep schedule. If you feel your energy draining constantly during the middle of your day, ask yourself what your sleep schedule is like. If it's pretty irregular, I would suggest first focusing on that. Taking a power nap when what your body really needs is consistent rest probably won't give you the results you are wanting. Healthy rest is more concerned about how well you rest than how much you rest.

If you do have a pretty regular sleep schedule but still feel you might need an extra boost in the middle of the day the power nap technique might be the place to start!

A few tips to start your power nap exercise are listed below.

- In the same way your body and mind will benefit most from a same time, same place mentality, so will your power nap. Find a space in your home, or anywhere that works, that you know will not be disturbed. If you work in the office everyday, don't be shy in taking a pillow and blanket into an empty office room and setting up shop. Of course, you may want to check with your employer but if it's only our lunch break, what can they say? If you know the office isn't where you're going to get any rest in, then try your car. It's quiet and no one, hopefully, will come knocking on your windows.

- 20 minutes is the preferred amount of time for a power nap. It gives you ample time for your brain to unwind, rest, and then come back to consciousness. You should feel energized post-nap, you want to make sure you're on top of your game going back into your day.

- Distractions will not be your friend. If you need to set your alarm on your phone, then make sure it's on silent once you press start. Shut down your computer and make sure you don't have anything too significant right after your nap. If you do, your brain may be more inclined to think of what is next than truly resting.

There are many tools you can lean into if you find yourself having trouble shutting your brain off and resting for 20 minutes in your day. There are apps for sleep noises and guided times of power naps. Whatever works best for you will be best for your body.

There are many ways to improve your sleep and rest routines. Routine is exactly the right word to use. The body thrives on structure, for the most part, and if you can get yourself to be in bed and wake up at relatively the same time each night and morning, you may see a big adjustment.

When your body and mind can rely on routine, it doesn't have to expect any coping mechanisms to come into play to overcompensate. Distractions and comfort are also great tools to keep in mind too. The lighter, hotter, and noisier your room, the less consistent sleep you will get. The best sleep environments are a dark room with little to no sound. Our bodies also do better in slightly colder temperatures for sleeping. So think about turning down your AC a few notches before you go to bed. You might want to have an extra comforter nearby, but that can help improve rest. The weight of blankets and comforters makes our minds relax and know we are safe and protected.

Diet is another component that can definitely amplify rest. When our bodies are ingesting lab-made chemicals, it goes through a lot more of a process to break down compounds and fully allow our bodies to digest. We all know sugar may taste good but it's not always the best for you. Natural sugars in fruits and vegetables are a healthy source of sugar. But others in candies or even non-whole-wheat breads or pastas can cause a lot of extra work for our bodies resulting in less rest and sleep.

Other foods can also be hard on the body when it comes to rest that aren't chemically made. Acidic foods like garlic, onions, and citric fruits can cause sleep deprivation. Alcohol can seem like it helps with sleep but just because it's easier to initially fall asleep doesn't mean it's the best right before bed. The alcohol has to be processed while we sleep so while you're snoozing away, your body is working overdrive. Many people tend to wake up in the middle of the night after having a night of alcohol. Either way, you may not wake up feeling refreshed and ready to give life your all if you're drinking some Jack and Cokes right before bed.

On top of keeping your health in check, physical exercise is great for sleeping. Toxins are released through the sweat and breath you expel while working out. Regularity in being physically active will definitely increase your sleep benefits. Head out on a long walk and examine the architecture in your neighborhood. Pump some iron at the gym or do your own circuit of exercises in your local park. High intensity workouts don't have to be the only way you get exercise. Swimming, aerobics, yoga, anything and everything that gets your body moving is nothing short of great work!

Many people don't prioritize sleep. Hasn't everyone heard someone say "I'll sleep when I'm dead"? How unhealthy! To have a fruitful and impactful practice of meditation rest is a necessity.

Chapter 5

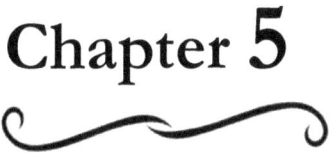

Tool Five:
Emotional Freedom Techniques (EFT) and Access Bars

*W*e've walked through meditation and the importance of resting your mind and heart. For some this may come easy. Relaxing by the pool and breathing in the fresh air. Pouring a slow cup of coffee as they watch rain wash down their driveway. But others... it may be a different story.

To take action in life means you are doing *something*. And a lot of people need to feel as though they are *doing* something to feel like they are accomplishing anything. Before jumping into this next chapter, I encourage you to take another moment to review the process you have been through with meditation and rest. Check your mind and align your heart. Are you jumping into the next chapter? Or have you sat with yourself and found solace in stillness? The answer to that question will only lead you back or forward. And there is no shame in either. Remember, acceptance is key. If stillness is hard for you, that is okay. But acknowledging what you are feeling is where you need to be.

If you are feeling ready and at rest then I invite you to continue on the path of the Law of Attraction.

Let's begin with what Emotional Freedom Techniques (EFT) even means. If you have had trouble in the past with the practice of manifestation, EFT may be where you need to be at this moment.

Resistance in one's life happens when they perceive they have failed. And if your practice at manifestation has brought you to the end of a rope then you may be having feelings of failure.

Resistance is anything that is not directly aligned with your inner self. It manifests itself as negative vibrations or things such as fear, anger, resentment, or anything that wears your mental capacity down.

This is exactly where EFT, or otherwise known as tapping, comes into play. When you don't know where to go in your practice of manifestation, tapping is the exact spot you should be.

Tapping

Tapping is an easy and simple practice and it will only take a few minutes out of your day.

1. Sit in a comfortable room that gives your mind and body space.

2. If you prefer, light a few incense, candles, or essential oils to merge your mind and body.

3. Keep a journal next to you of the issue at hand i.e. ―I cannot attract my career" or ―Ican't move past this emotional block."

4. On a different piece of paper write down affirmations towards yourself that you will repeat throughout the process.

5. Find a few different pressure points you can easily access.

6. Begin tapping these points. While you tap, keep in mind your block while repeating out loud to yourself the affirmations you wrote down.

Have fun with the process and let your mind release the negative vibrations into the air. This practice only takes a few minutes to see results.

Here is a list of a few limiting beliefs your subconscious may be holding on to:

- I am not allowed to succeed
- I am not loved
- I am not valued
- No one wants me
- I have to do X for someone to receive Y for myself

Here is a list of affirmations you can repeat to yourself:

- I have capabilities that no one else has
- I am known
- I am loved
- I am allowed to set boundaries for my own personal well-being
- I am worthy

On top of this practice being fulfilling, there are a few tips to keep in mind when practicing:

- Drink plenty of water—Water not only flushes out toxins from food and liquids but also from deeper within. Drink plenty of water to release toxins from all corners of your body.

- Stay consistent—If you are a morning person, great! Incorporate the art of tapping into your morning routine. Sit down with a cup of coffee and hash out all those negative vibes!

- Continue to be persistent—The practice may not release every negative thought or resistance you have in your body the first or second time. It may take time and that is totally okay! Remember to be persistent in the practice and continue giving yourself that self-love through the process.

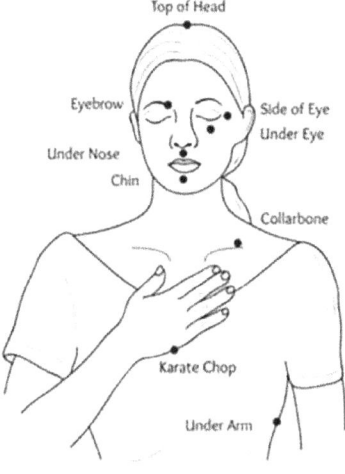

EFT Tapping Points

Access Bars

Your brain holds a lot of power within your body. It's the lifesource for decision-making, emotions, body movement, and so much more. With so much power inside an organ, there has to be things that aren't supposed to be there as well.

This is where the 32 access bars come into play. There are 32 energy bars that run through your brain and they all connect to different aspects of your life.

Awareness	Control	Creativity	Life Forms
Manifestation	Kindness	Power	Aging
Body	Re-Creation	Crown	Creation

Sexuality	Re-Activation	Sadness	Time
Space	Joy	Reconstructing	Implant
Communication	Healing	Form	Structure
Hope	Gratitude	Peace	Calm
Dreams	Prosperity		

When you invest in a session to align your access bars, you will be releasing all the trapped self-doubt and negative thoughts your brain holds. Whether you are conscious of these thoughts or not, your brain knows they are there. When a trained professional lays you down for an access bar session, they will be touching each bar. When touching each bar, the gentle pressure will release electromagnetic charges that hold negative emotions within.

Do you feel like you can't get past a certain negative emotion? Have you felt angry? Or sad?

When was the last time you felt yourself completely relaxed without worry or expectations hanging on the edge of your consciousness?

The best place to receive a 32 bar access therapy session is by a professional in your area. It takes time and dedication to know where each energy bar is on your scalp so make sure your therapist is well equipped.

If you feel access bar therapy might not work for you, at least give it a try and at the very least you'll experience an amazing scalp massage.

Chapter 6

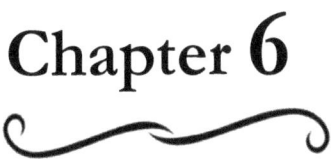

Tool Six:
Harmony, Right Action, and Moving Your Body

Harmony

The Law of Attraction can be used to bring material goods and desires into your grasp but as we have walked through previously, it can also help you manifest the inner well-being of your mind and heart. Harmony has many different meanings but essentially all the definitions blend together in a... let's say, harmonious way. When you think of an instrument what might come to mind are a few chords. They all are played at the same time and ring together with a sort of effortlessness. Some people find music to be such a part of their core that it brings about transformations just by a tune or a note. When a band plays all sorts of instruments, if they're good, it will sound beautiful. The chords may bring up different memories, emotions, or strong desires towards someone or something. In a strictly instrumental definition, this would be considered harmony. What if you aren't playing instruments? The same idea can be applied to your inner life as well as your outer one.

When you focus on harmony in your life, you will receive and acknowledge what you truly believe is important and a priority to you. Have you ever noticed that things continue to come your way that may not be ideal? Have you thought about the balances in your life? Do you have an estranged relative where things ended on bad terms? Have you disrupted the balance of someone else's life by meddling or gossiping? Take a look at your inner life. How are your practices in meditation going? Do you feel anger or hate towards an event that happened to you? The harmony we have towards others and the harmony we have towards ourselves can all be intertwined with what the Universe is giving and taking.

If you do find yourself analyzing and realizing there are things in your life out of harmony or balance, that is a great first step into helping the problem. I would suggest going into a time of meditation or beginning your practice. Start with a full body and mind scan. Acknowledge where harmony is not aligned and release it. If this means taking physical actions, do so.

When harmony enters your life, you can enjoy your career, your relationships, your financial status because you won't have unbalanced emotions interfering with your life.

Let's break down some actions you can take to step into a life of harmony.

In the words of Gandhi;

—Happiess is when what you think, what you say, and what you do are all in harmony."

To effectively incorporate harmony into your life and utilize it in the mindset of the Law of Attraction, it really begins with your mindset.

Like I said early, everyone in life has had hardships. Insignificant to others or surmounting to all, challenges are a part of life. How we view these challenges and how we walk towards healing is all about our perspective. To be human is to be born into pain, disappointments, and hard lessons but to say that life is simply pain is completely wiping away a whole other side of what it is to be alive. Of course, I can't sit here and take ownership for what life has thrown at you. But I can say I am truly sorry for whatever you have faced. I encourage you to continue reading and seek to find the beauty in life.

To bring harmony is to accept, heal, and believe we are able to overcome. And not only overcome but choose to believe what has happened to us has only made us stronger to take on life and laugh in adversity.

The one who is able to appreciate the life they were dealt and look on it with even a faint smile is someone who has taken hold of harmony within themselves.

Of course we all envision the perfect life. That car, job, partner, animal, or body but harmony isn't all about attracting the material goods in your life to yourself. Like before, harmony is embracing what you have and being content in where you are now.

Positivity is key. It may be a cliche but it's a good one. It's so easy to point to the negative, the painful, the thing that didn't go your way. Instead of sitting in the negative, take a moment to focus on the positive. View yourself from outside of where you are, outside of the situation and analyze it from a different perspective. You might see some things aren't as bad as they might feel at the moment.

Daily meditation is a game-changer. To sit with yourself and allow space and time to hear, see, and acknowledge yourself will do wonders for your inner harmonious life. Center yourself, regain focus and gratitude. Meditation will allow you to take ownership and control over emotions and may help you see not all is bad.

What does harmony look like to you? Maybe creating a vision board once a day will help you center your focus and remember what harmony means to you. There are thousands of examples of what this could look like depending on the person. A picture of the ocean. Not a swimmer? What about vast mountains with lush green ivy? You could put a picture up of a balanced meal, encouraging health and mindfulness for your food. A family picture could promote harmony or a best friend. Again, it's all based on who you are. There are no right or wrong ways to visualize harmony for yourself.

Remove stressors from your life. To focus on harmony, it does take practice and dedication. There are probably stressors in your life that do exactly the opposite. A friend that has toxic behaviors? Is it technology? Set aside a time each day for you to put your phone away and be present. Family can be a stressors for many people; potentially look into what healthy boundaries may look like for you in that area of your life.

The Law of Right Action

The Law of Right Action goes hand-in-hand with the Law of Attraction. Essentially, the Law of Right Action tells us to take responsibility for what we do, say, think, desire, even for the quality of our life. The main basis for this law is to take responsibility for who you are and what you do. Without giving ourselves value, how are we able to give value to others around us? The Law of Right Action pushes us to take steps towards practices that will enhance our own self-value so we can rightly see others and acknowledge their worth. If you choose, or have chosen, to not take actions towards ownership or bringing balance to yourself, then the Law of Right Action would claim it is on your shoulders.

To acknowledge and believe that strength and empowerment will only come from within yourself is the best place to start with right action. If you value yourself then others will have to follow your lead in how they treat you. Again, it all starts with you. Tactfulness is a great skill to have when stepping into the Law of Right Action. If others are complaining, misdirecting ownership, or causing major damage to their inner well-being, it's probably best to handle them with care. You can easily tell someone the hard truth without care for their emotions or feelings but that would be acting directly against right action. First, begin with yourself and then gradually you will be able to guide people towards actions for themselves in their own life.

—No blaming and no excuses!" It's easy to say but pretty hard to incorporate into your life. What if a car almost clips you on the side of the road? It was their fault! They weren't even watching. Or were you on your phone and walking blindly? To live without excuses is a hard task to take on but you might find it frees you from so much.

Another form of right action is to live in balance. Some may struggle with self-absorption while others may only see the needs of the people around them. Neither of these extremes are healthy. To live in balance is to adequately serve yourself and to also know others have pains and struggles as much as you do. It may take time to find this balance and what is best and healthiest for you but the Law of Right Action will only reward you for your hardwork and ownership.

Have you often found yourself saying phrases like ‗life is the worst', or ‗there is truly no point to life'. The Law of Right Action would say in response to you, ―Well, what are you going to do about it?". You have the power to change your life. You have the authority to quit the job you hate, end the relationship that's draining, move cities. You can and if you truly want change, you will. Ask yourself some hard questions. Do you want to succeed in change? Or do you quietly enjoy your life how it is; the routine, the same friends, the neighborhood. It can be hard to answer honestly because as human beings, we are prone to not like change. So maybe if you find yourself answering no to changing things in your life, you aren't quite ready *to* change. If that is the case, you may need to spend some time in meditation to release those negative thoughts and emotions.

I would challenge you to break apart the illusions that your life may suck if you find yourself repeating that phrase over and over again. Do you find your life unsatisfying because you are comparing yourself to others around you? Is life hard because you haven't been able to nail that job you've been working towards for so long? These are all thoughts that block you from your fullest potential. Remember earlier when we talked about your mind not knowing lack unless you are giving it something to lack? This is exactly where you need to bring the practice of the Law of Attraction into play. Release all these hindering thoughts and emotions and begin living where you are. Embrace yourself and those around you and rid yourself of comparison and envy.

Moving Your Body

Harmony and the Law of Right Action both boil down to the act of movement. Harmony is the act of doing the hard work of self-acceptance and giving to others what you yourself have received. The Law of Right Action is about putting life into action. Many different forms and styles play a part in moving your body. It doesn't have to mean a long run or lifting weights. It could mean moving your body into action of your plans, hopes, and desires.

It also means accepting yourself as who and what you are. Find a practice of moving your body that works best with who you are and go from there. It isn't about getting it right the first time but giving yourself grace and patience in the process. Maybe start with some daily stretches, or implement a plan to get something done within a few days. Whatever it is, it's your journey and it's worth taking.

Chapter 7

The 12 Laws of the Universe

So much revolves around the Law of Attraction and all the ways you can incorporate it into your own life to get where you want to go. It may shock you to find out there are other universal laws that play a major part in the world and life around you. Although, the Law of Attraction is a great law to start with and brings deeper understanding too, it might be helpful to know there are 11 other universal laws. Depending on your own life and what you deem as necessary and important in your own life will dictate which law may be best for you to study next, but I'll map out the 11 other laws for you below.

The Law of Divine Oneness

The Law of Divine Oneness specifically speaks to the idea, or knowledge, that everything is connected. Some person you pass, every event you experience, everything you do is all connected to one another and to the lives around you. Some claim this law is the one that connects all the rest together. Which makes sense if the fundamental idea of this law is exactly that: oneness. There is a phrase that backs this rule which is called the ‗hive mind'. The hive mind claims when we all act and react to one another as if we truly believe I am connected to you in the same way you are connected to me, then there would be more understanding and compassion for humanity. To have one purpose, motive, and action is to have one mind or a hive mind. Think of a colony of bees, they each do their work throughout the day. They don't all pollinate at one flower or else that flower will not have any further use to the bees. They also don't follow each other from one bunch of flowers to the next. They each, on their own, do as they know is best for the colony by spreading out to different parts of a forest or area to gain as much pollination for their collective family. Think of the human race in the same way. We may not all be on the same path as each other, each going to the same restaurants, jobs, or countries but if we believe we are all one in the same there would be a better collective truth.

That is not to say we all need to have the same opinions and beliefs. If that were the case, individualism would go out the door. No, instead of believing we all need to act and be the same, it's the understanding of the truth that what I do affects you and what you do affects me. If I truly believe we are of one mind, then when I hurt or insult you what I am truly doing is shining those repercussions onto myself. It's a mutual respect and love for one another. This also doesn't just quit at the people or lives around you but everything you interact with. Every thought, event, or action you take is interconnected to all other lives. To hurt the Earth is to directly inflict pain onto yourself and humanity.

If you believe that you are not worth life, don't deserve certain things, or simply hold onto negative things within yourself like anger, frustration, resentment, or anything else, that inherently negatively impacts the whole of the hive. What I mean is if you hold resentment towards yourself or towards someone else, those emotions and negative vibrations will inevitably reach back out to others you don't mean to inflict pain into. Because your vibrations are constantly reverberating off of you and into others, what you feel and experience is what the collective whole experiences and feels. That is why it is so important to go through the work we discussed in the previous chapters, it holds such importance for not only yourself but for the hive mind around you.

Collective meditation is a wonderful way to bring a group of people into positive vibrations that will enhance the group narrative. Many people are unaware they are holding negative vibrations within themselves, or if they do they might not be aware of how deep those vibrations go. To meditate with others around you, all at once you are releasing those negative emotions and welcoming in positivity as a whole. How beneficial that is for humanity and the Earth if we could all learn to embrace one another as ourselves. Also, if you take the time to work through healing your own mind, how beneficial would that be for the people in your sphere when they come into contact with you? If you are working and succeeding in healing your mind, those vibrations will only help the ones you are around to heal as well.

A few tips on how to practice the Law of Divine Oneness is to incorporate it into your own meditation time. This could mean while on your own you take breaths to acknowledge the people and things around you. Take some time to find a few people you know. Maybe even stretch yourself to a few people that aren't your favorite to be around. We definitely all have those people whether they are irritating or unjustly wronged us. Once you have a few in your inner being, take a few deep breaths and recognize who they are. Bring into mind how you met, what your conversations are about, and how they might need an extension of compassion from you. Acknowledge these people are, in fact, closer to you than you might have realized before. As you breathe out, let go of negativity towards them and breathe in understanding.

Another way to practice this law is to interact with nature in a way that honors who she is. Sit in the woods and breathe in her fresh breath and out the toxicity that comes with being human. Accept her as an entity that brings about pureness and allow her positive vibrations to seep into your inner being. There are so many ways you can practice mindfulness of being One with everything and anything around you but the main point is to extend compassion.

The Law of Vibration

We talked briefly about the Law of Vibration but it plays a bigger role in understanding the universe than a brief interlude of explanation. To simply define what the Law of Vibration is to explain that everything and everyone has a vibration frequency. At a small level, microscopic, everything vibrates. Chairs, desks, the floor your feet may be on, everything has a frequency rate that we may or may not be able to feel but this extends past the physical into the spiritual as well. Our frequency of vibrations informs our own reality. Based on what our vibrations are giving off to the world results in what we receive from the world.

A great example of the Law of Vibration is to talk about money. You may be getting bonuses and checks from work because you are bringing the positive vibrations you focus on and practice with into your workplace. But you might be noticing you aren't able to hang on to that frequency of money. Perhaps you gamble it away once you receive it, maybe you accidentally crash your car and that extra bonus you just received has to be put to use for something very practical. Or maybe you even experienced someone robbing you and all that extra hard work was taken away from you. There may be a cause and effect situation you might not be able to understand but it may also have to do with your own practice of vibration frequency. The higher the vibrations within ourselves the more positive outcomes and effects we will experience. The lower vibrations we have, the more negative outcomes we will experience in life. Another way you can phrase the Law of Vibration is by saying it is the frequency of your energy.

Someone's energy isn't something you can feel or see with your eyes but something you can sense and react to. The idea behind this law is to learn you have the ability to change your frequency and adjust it when certain circumstances require it. The vibrations you hold within yourself affect your entire being. There are a few ways you can learn to manage and grow in learning how to adjust your vibrations.

We've talked through manifestation but in order to receive something you are aiming to achieve, you have to know how to match your vibrations to that certain thing. Again, if you are wanting to have more money and that is what you are focusing on, your subconscious mind will cling to what you are lacking thus resulting in a lower, negative frequency of vibrations. To direct your own thoughts toward things that are plentiful and hold gratitude results in achieving those positive vibes.

To be able to tap into what you are sensing at any given time based on the vibrations around you is a great tool to stretch and master. By being able to understand what you are feeling and how those environments or people are either positively or negatively affecting your inner vibrations you will then be able to decide who and what situations are good for you. If you continually walk into a restaurant but while eating there you notice your mind turning towards what you lack or feelings of anxiety, be self-aware enough to recognize that the atmosphere is surrounded with negative vibrations. Once you are able to sense what people, places, things, or activities have higher vibrations, you will be able to discern and sense when you are around those vibrations in everyday life.

Emotions are also a great indicator in how to manage our vibrational frequency. If you find yourself feeling angry or frustrated, it's best to recognize that. Once you have acknowledged those emotions and accepted you are feeling something negative like anger then it is time to go into self-reflection or meditation. This will help because emotions are a gateway into our hearts. If we are feeling angry over a situation or person it is a good indicator we are either harboring deeper negative vibrations we weren't aware of or that event or person needs to have boundaries around it for us to feel safer. To feel anger or negative emotions is not a bad thing, it is actually very beneficial. But how we respond and react to those emotions is what plays into our overall well-being of our vibrational frequencies.

Oftentimes, we are taught there are good and bad emotions, this is simply not true. All it means is that we need to recognize and take the right steps to work through what we feel and release them. This will help you not feel the weight of those emotions and will also grow your vibrations into a higher frequency.

Another way to raise your vibrations to a higher frequency is to take into account your diet and lifestyle. Obviously, heavy, unhealthy foods will not help our bodies feel nourished and be able to do the work that needs to be done to focus on our inner being. Take some time and maybe start a food log. Write down what you eat during your week. How much sugar intake? What about the amount of water you're allowed to come into your body? Our bodies need to be nurtured as much as our minds do and it can help immensely with our frequencies.

It may be hard to distinguish the difference between the Law of Vibration and the Law of Attraction. If you are asking that question, it makes total sense. The difference between the two may not be bountiful but it is significant.

The Law of Vibration is all about matching the frequency of what we are pursuing whether that be a relationship, job, or life change. The Law of Attraction takes that one step further by saying you have the ability to create within yourself the frequency necessary to achieve the frequency you are looking for. Essentially, the Law of Vibration leads directly into the Law of Attraction in saying that what you are in alignment with vibrationally will manifest with better ease.

The Law of Correspondence

The Law of Correspondence is very unique in that it states the patterns we have seen before repeat themselves throughout the universe. In the same way our personal lives are a reflection of what is happening within ourselves. There is a saying by Hermes Trismegistus that goes; —Asabove, so below. As within, so without." This is the essence of the Law of Correspondence. What is happening within us will reflect what happens outside of us.

If you are dealing with low self-esteem and you look in the mirror every day and hate what you see, that will only reflect into your life on the outside too. What I mean is if you hate how you look and then later that day you walk into a meeting, your low self-esteem will inevitably be reflected in your presentation. Your boss may be thinking, ─I don't know why he's acting like this. Some weeks he's ready to get work done while others he's just barely here." Your boss is picking up on your inner being and he knows, whether consciously or not, what you are feeling within is what he is seeing without.

Here is another example; if you are getting drinks with a group of people you don't truly enjoy, what you feel towards them within your mind will only come out in conversation and action. That group of people may even be able to pick up on what you are feeling and how you are acting and confront you about it. You may not have even noticed that you dislike this group of people but now you are faced with either telling the truth to yourself and those friends or to keep it hidden.

Our thoughts and actions that we have in our conscious mind subconsciously extend to our outer world. If we try to change our external circumstances but have not confronted our internal mind, then what we hold within ourselves will only continue to be a part of our external world. If you decide to move away from the city you live in because of a falling out with family but refuse to interact with your inner mind, when you move to the next city it is only a matter of time until those same actions and words reappear in your ‚new life'. To change your mindset is to change your reality. But, as we've discussed, changing your mindset takes a lot of discipline and desire. But I believe in you and know you have the inner strength to do so.

Unless you start taking responsibility for your thoughts and face the demons inside yourself you will continue to live in a victim mindset. There are some things we cannot control. And I guarantee there are people reading this who had horrible events happen to them that were completely outside their control. It's heartbreaking and again, I am sorry. But to break free from the control that others or the world has had over you is beautiful and groundbreaking. Start taking more responsibility for your micro-world and you will begin to notice changes in your macro-world.

There are practical steps you can take to change your inner world so it will reflect in your outer world. Below is a list of actions and reactions that may help you change those lower frequencies.

- When someone negatively speaks to or about you, speak gently back to them.

- When you are in pain or hurting, show someone else extra love and compassion.

- If you feel useless or unworthy, communicate encouragement to someone else.

- When you are in fear or afraid, send comfort to someone through your presence or thoughts.

When you react to actions that logically feel like they deserve negative energies, you are changing the dynamic of your life. You are healing the part of yourself that has been wounded in your past and, thus, progressing and moving towards a more full, whole, and positive life.

Think of the example of floating down a river on a raft. The waters are calm, drifting you side to side, the cold water is hitting you just when the sun becomes a little too hot. It's calm, peaceful, and your mind is relaxed. Now some time passes and you start to hear rapids ahead of you. Immediately, your mind and body both react to those rapids. Usually in that type of situation you will try and take control of every aspect of what is about to happen to you. You may forcibly paddle backwards or sideways which would result in overturning your raft. But if you allow your body and mind to succumb to the flow of the waters it would be easier to make it through the rapids safely. In your outer world when you feel a jolt in life, take some time to reflect inward and process through why there may be a disconnection between your inner mind and your outer body.

The Law of Attraction

The Law of Attraction is the next law of the universe in line, but since all you have heard previously is based on this law I suspect we don't need to go any further in depth.

To sum up all that we have talked about previously into a simplified statement, the Law of Attraction is the fact that like attracts like. You obtain what you focus and aim for in life. If you are wanting love but aren't willing to give love to others, your subconscious inner mind will only give to you more of what you are lacking.

The Law of Right Action

The Law of Right Action is also very similar to the Law of Attraction and also one we briefly touched on previously. To bring all we have discussed into a summary is to say the Law of Right Action is truly about taking *real* action in your life. To simply meditate, think, or desire something won't really get you to where you want to go. There is a portion of your life that has to be put into action. As we spoke previously, to begin this law it is all about sitting with yourself and discerning what the best and next step for you needs to be. This can be done through meditation, journaling, hiking, or any other number of ways. But what has to come out of this inner reflection is a plan of action. A key factor of this law is to not have your fists closed. To be open to all and any possibilities will yield the best results for you and your life.

The Law of Perpetual Transmutation of Energy

That's a long title with a lot of longer words... So what does this law actually mean? Well, let's break down what each word is defined as.

Perpetual is something that never stops.

Transmutation is just a big word for changing the state of something.

And energy... well energy is everything that is in and around us.

So, to simplify this law of the universe it's pretty much saying that everything around us is always changing and will never stop changing. To take the understanding of this law a step further is to say that we have the ability to change the energies that are always around us. Pretty cool, right?

Everything is moving. All things are evolving and fluctuating and constantly in motion. On a very basic level, a tree sprout continues to grow as the sun hits its leaves. When the tree is at its fullest capacity of growth, then it produces fruit or nuts or continually grows new leaves. A baby is born as a small, defenseless being and over the course of it's life continues to grow until one day it's body gives up. Everything evolves and moves into something that it wasn't the previous day. But of course, this law doesn't just stop at the physical aspects of life. Our minds, spirits, souls, inner thoughts and being continue to transform and grow even if someone does not do the hard work of self-actualization. Whether you are growing towards a fuller and whole self or feel as though you are stagnant in your life, you are still evolving. It just depends on whether you are moving towards a healthier being or an unhealthier one.

The basis for this law is that everything is energy. Our thoughts and emotions become actions. Every thought, every feeling has energy behind it and that energy is then transferred into an energy of action.

Because our thoughts become our actions, this requires a baseline of consistency in our intentions.

If our thoughts are inconsistent and rapidly changing, the universe will have a hard time sending anything our way besides erratic vibrations and energies. Change is necessary and will always happen in life but the more consistent we are with ourselves and our thoughts, the more consistent we will receive energy from the universe. It all comes back to being honest with yourself and taking the right steps to work through areas in your inner being that are in alignment with each other. If you are desiring love your subconscious will discern that you are actually lacking love. Also, if you are desiring love but only have feelings of unworthiness and low self-esteem, those energies are very jumbled and the universe will not truly know your intentions.

To transfer energy from within yourself to your outer world it is necessary to focus on your goals and thoughts in a positive understanding and then stick to the knowledge that what energies you give to the world will return to you. When this is being done, there is finally consistency from within yourself and the energies you are giving out. Energy is always wanting to manifest itself into physical attributes or situations.

It may be hard to know how to transfer your negative energy into something that is positive in your outer world. Let's say you are grieving a situation that happened. Perhaps a family pet passed away recently or you lost your job. Turn the sad, negative energy into something that brings positivity to the world. Take time to create something. Maybe you enjoy painting and know you can process your emotions of grief through buying paints and canvases. Creating something out of negative energy is a great way to transfer your inner energy into a positive outer energy. How about you feeling angry about something. A friend stood you up on a night you were meant to get drinks. Or you had an argument with a family member. Take that negative energy you are experiencing and flush it out into positive outcomes. You could go on a run, take a boxing class, or just workout. Those negative emotions are sure to come out into the world through a more positive light like helping your health.

Just know if you don't find a way for your internal negative energy to come out through a path that will create positive external energy, then that negativity will come out another way. It's better to take control of what you are feeling rather than an unexpected outburst of anger or frustration being released into your outer world.

Keep in mind that you are always growing towards more life or more death. It sounds intense but it's true. You can either embrace and accept this law of the universe or fight against it and allow the unexpected and possibly harmful results to affect your life.

To state or claim that what you are and what you have is unchangeable is simply untrue. If you don't like the relationship you're in, change it. If you don't like the diet you're on, change it. Your hair? Change it. You have the ability and the opportunity to change the energy that is around you into something else! Into anything else.

You may be asking yourself a few questions though and they may sound like this; "I'm poor. I live from one paycheck to another. Of course I want to be wealthier. Of course I want to have more flexibility with my money and resources. Are you saying that all I have to do to get rich is change my mindset?"

The answer to the question is yes! Just change your mindset. Sounds really easy. And your reply may be something in the zone if you have done that for years. Why would you want to be poor? Why would you want to not have enough money to do anything else besides pay bills? It comes down to your inner, subconscious mindset. Many people who want to be wealthier have only ever known the financial status they are currently in. You may have seen some fluctuations in status of class but you probably are around the same money intake as you were given as a child. The trick is what your mind is thinking, even subconsciously. You probably think and believe that you are poor. Because you are so focused on how poor you actually are, you will continue to stay in that subconscious mindset. I'm not saying to blow all your money on ice cream and new clothes. No, not at all. But I am saying you can change the energies of your mind. If you believe that what you have is abundance and wealth, then your status of life will become one of abundance and wealth.

If you had no concept of poverty then your thoughts wouldn't revolve around it. You would think that your world is full, abundant, and wealthy. You have the power to bring that into fruition. You have the capacity to change your life! It may sound cheesy but it's true; you just have to believe you can.

The Law of Cause and Effect

Every action will have a reaction. We've all heard this in science class right? That is the basic understanding of the Law of Cause and Effect. Makes sense and it is one of the most straightforward laws we will talk about. Beginning at a cosmic level, it's important to understand that every effect first had a cause. The creation of the world, the beginning of life on earth, the start of your career all had a beginning cause. From those first causes there is a chain reaction of effects that span into many different avenues. There could be thousands of offshoots that come from one cause in your life, one beginning. In line with this law it is believed that every action, step, or decision you make has a cosmic effect that reaches past yourself.

Everything is interconnected. You cannot make a movement or a decision without affecting something near or around you. When you take a step, you are moving the space that your leg is touching thus reacting to ripple effects throughout the universe that you may not be able to see or understand. We are all interconnected and react to the universe around us whether we know it or not. And same goes for the universe's reaction to our actions. Everything that has existed once came from the same, at some point throughout history, microscopic beginning.

Bringing this law to a more macro level, human thought brings around a reaction whether we are sitting still or walking throughout the city. When you are thinking, there is inevitable action. This may look like a physical action; I am thinking about coffee so I take action to get coffee. Or it may shine through in simple behaviors; I am thinking about how my boss screwed me over so I will ignore him this week.

According to this law, there is an understanding that nothing happens by chance.

Everything that happens to or from you came from an intentional action or behavior that has then reflected onto you or those around you.

Let's break this down a bit.

Say you are walking by a building and something falls at your feet. You can trace that action to a reaction of something else. Maybe a bird knocked that object off the ledge accidentally. Maybe a person threw it out the window. Whatever that initial action was, there was a first action that caused all the ripple effects. That bird, for some reason, decided it wanted more room to sit on the windowsill thus knocking off the object to land in front of you. Or that person decided they would rather throw that object out the window than walk to their trash can to throw it away. Whatever it was, there was a first action. And those actions from the bird or the person then had even further beginning actions that had to take place. Because of this series of events it creates a bond between your physical or mental space and the action that first started it. You are interconnected and unable to separate from the eternal state of cause and effect in life.

The Law of Cause and Effect has been called many different things. Some determine it to be the same as karma. The simple understanding of karma is what I do will come back to me. Whether that be in a negative light or a positive one. Either way your actions will cause a reaction. Or, you reap what you sow. Many Buddhists and Hindus believe that the universe takes into account your intentions behind the actions.

Say you bring someone a present. You wrap it for them and present it as something they should love and admire. But deep in your inner consciousness you know the present you are about to give them won't be something they will actually love or want. You've given them the gift out of the intention of spite rather than good nature. The universe will see that energy and the reaction to your action will probably be a negative one.

Many get caught up in the immediacy of this law though. You may expect that because you have done something good you should or will receive the reaction within the next few hours. This concept is a misinterpretation of the law. It would be hard to distinguish which reaction came from which action you performed. Years ago you may have done something out of good intent and today the universe has rippled it back into your life. That isn't to say that what you did yesterday is the cause of what you have received today.

Mindfulness is such a great practice and as I hope you have noticed, is paramount to the practice of the Law of Attraction. But it also plays a major role in the Law of Cause and Effect. The more mindful you are with your choices, actions, and behaviors, the deeper your awareness will be of the effects of your decisions. The best way you can practice mindfulness is by being brutally honest with yourself. No lies, no deceitfulness, no victim mindset. Take your actions and your behaviors for what they are and when you notice yourself reacting in a negative way to circumstances, make the change that is necessary. You have that power. Understand that your thoughts are most likely the most primary cause of your outer world. Once you are able to take control of your inner thoughts and life, your outer world will fall into line as well.

The Law of Compensation

In changing moon, in tidal wave,

Glows the feud of Want and Have.

Gauge of more and less through space

Electric star and pencil plays.

The lonely Earth amid the balls

That hurry through the eternal halls,

A makeweight flying to the void,

Supplemental asteroid,

Or compensatory spark,

Shoots across the neutral Dark.

—Ralph Waldo Emerson

Emerson wrote a dissertation on his views and ideas of the Law of Compensation. Although his words may be lofty and a bit hard to decipher if you aren't used to pulling apart poetry, he understands the concept of this universal law. Emerson states that every day, as the moon changes its phases, the human heart continues to feel a pull between what we want and what we have.

Other people are prone to call this law of the universe the law of behavior. Its basis is similar to the Law of Attraction but it tends to ask you to take a bit more responsibility for your efforts and actions. It states that no matter how much effort you put into your practice of life, you will be compensated for any amount of it. In life there will always be action and for every action, there will be a reaction.

You may be thinking about your job. It's easy to associate this law with work. Since at work you may get paid based on how much effort you put in. That's a great comparison but it doesn't stop there and it doesn't necessarily depend on money. If you spend your time sending love and giving love to others it may make sense to you that you would then receive love back. But the law doesn't state that what you put effort into you will have returned to you in the same manner. It does state that if you put effort into giving love, you will be compensated for that love. It may be in love being returned to you but it also may look like finances, hope, provision. This law doesn't state you will get what you give in the exact manner but that your efforts in life will be compensated.

Take some time and spend it thinking about all you have contributed and made an effort in life for. Have you raised children? That takes a lot of effort. How has the universe compensated you? It may look like a loving relationship with your child or children. Happiness in your partner. A job that you love? Or maybe you haven't felt like you received compensation yet. It will come. Or maybe you could spend some more time realizing what you have been compensated for already.

If you don't put the effort into life then there can also be diminishing compensations as well. We've talked a lot about the vibrations you hold within yourself. If you withhold those from the world, it will notice. In the same way we think about our work space, it relates to this law as well. If you don't decide to put in effort, happiness, gratitude, or energy then there will be nothing to show for it. To overcome or avoid diminishing compensation, come to a point in your life where you aren't doing things to get things. Truly seek to love others without expectations for more wealth or happiness. Learn to put in effort and passion into your life without just expecting a return and a reward.

Your compensation is a direct correlation to the value of effort you put into your actions and life. The key word there is value. If you head over to your local soup kitchen and are there so you will be given your dream car or a raise you want but your heart's not in a loving state, you will be compensated based on the value of the work there. You could be there, helping feed the homeless but instead of acting in love you're throwing the food onto their plate, counting down the minutes until you can leave, and not making eye contact. The value of your work will be compensated, not simply your actions. If you give more than expected, your compensation will increase. If you give more than you believe you are able, your compensation will increase.

If you spend your day focusing your energy and thoughts on gratitude, happiness, joy, and love in return you will be given gratitude, happiness, joy, and love. The result of your efforts in desiring a happier life for you will be compensated in a deeper awareness of what you do have in life. In the contrasting sense, if you are focusing on how much you hate people, your job, your family, and life then you will be compensated with exactly those things. Our minds are such powerful tools and in the same way the Christian Bible states, "take captive every thought", it is essential you decide what you want out of your life and how you decide to think about life is what can help impact the most out of the Law of Compensation.

The Law of Relativity

Everything is neutral. We may be tempted to compare things in our life but the reality, based on this law, is that everything is neutralized within life. Have you ever heard that the thief of joy is the act of comparison? This law speaks directly to that inclination we all have.

The definition of relativity is stated as the absence of standards.

If you happen to live in Alaska you then know that it is dark for a portion of the year and light for the rest. You also know that temperatures on average in the summer are around 60 degrees fahrenheit. To someone who is from Georgia, that sounds like autumn or spring. If you both were to get together and compare and contrast your summer temperatures, you both would think the other was living in either extreme heat or cold for summer days. Your truth to your life is relative on many factors. A simple example is the temperatures at where you live but this law goes far beyond just temperatures.

The Law of Relativity can help increase compassion for everyone. It's hard to distinguish why people believe and think what they believe and think. It may help if you sit down with someone and give them the time to talk through their life experiences but even then you didn't live their life or feel the things that impacted them. If you pass someone on the street who is acting in a protest of some sort that you don't agree with or understanding, think about putting the Law of Relativity into practice. You may not agree with what they are advocating for but those people have a reason and a purpose that goes deeper than what is seen.

Let's put the easier example into context. Say you are one side of the political sphere and you pass a protest that is advocating for the other side of your political ideologies. You may not understand why they would take the time to stand outside for hours, holding heavy signs, and asking for a reform in the government's law. But what if after the protest was over you asked one of those protestors to get coffee with you. While you're sitting down drinking your coffee, you get into the conversation of why that person feels so inclined towards their political sphere. You end up getting to have the opportunity to hear their beliefs, their passions, their hurts, and pains and why all of those things are incorporated into them making the decision to protest. You may not still be able to say you would switch political sides but at least you can exercise the Law of Relativity and have compassion over the person you're sharing a table with. To accept and understand that that person has different circumstances than you is to extend compassion towards them. In the opposite sense, you could have walked by the crowd of protestors and gone to work to slander the bigots that blindly make the wrong decision to support a group that is 'wrong'. To sit and assess someone else's decisions without applying the Law of Relativity is to withhold understanding and compassion. The outcome to that decision is to only expect the same reactions towards you and your life.

To not accept and apply the Law of Relativity when you are faced with adversity is then to attract and hold within lower frequencies of vibrations. This will only bring about negativity into your life. To extend understanding and gratitude for that person or idea you oppose is to bring about a higher frequency of positive vibrations into your life.

An easier example to use for this law is again about temperature. If you set your house to the temperature of 65 degrees, many would say that it is very cold. But if you walk outside in winter and experience the 15 degree coldness of December and then come back inside to the 65 degree house, it will be warmer to you. It's relative.

The Law of Polarity

Everything has an opposite. Love, apathy. Excitement, disappointment. A warm shower and a cold one. This law is all about understanding and accepting that everything has an opposite. To use this law is to understand how to bring a good thing out of what may seem bad.

If you are going through a horrible breakup, think about it in a polar opposite sense. If you're heartbroken and your true love left you without explanation allow yourself to see it from the opposite view. That person probably wasn't extending love to you in the same way you were or in the way you needed. As much as it hurts to accept, and as easy it is to say than put into practice, it may be a blessing that at first looks like a curse. If you are able to unlock this understanding, you may be able to unlock some blocks within your inner life. And maybe you do look at the opposite of what you were given and you decide that it still sucks and that it wasn't beneficial. At least acknowledge that any type of contrast brings about a clarity you might not have had before.

The best example for the Law of Polarity is to bring the image of a battery into your mind. I'm sure most of us had those science classes where we were taught about circuits. And if not, at least we've had enough experience with batteries to know there is a positive and negative end. When hooking up batteries from one to another you have to make sure they are all flowing in the same direction or else the chain of energy will not be able to flow. That connection can either be in a negative fluid motion or a positive. If you want to add more batteries to the line of energy, again they all have to align in the same exact form or else it won't work. The Law of Polarity suggests that many people want to use more batteries but set them up in the opposite directions. Instead of having two batteries facing the same way, there's a confusion of which battery needs to sit which way and the flow of energy is disrupted.

To use the Law of Polarity to your benefit and for your intentions takes some inner work. Surprise, surprise! But again, all this inner work will definitely benefit you. After you've done that inner work with yourself and are able to identify your *true* intentions on what you are after, all you have to do is be consistent with those intentions. To one day be content in your work and then the next abhor your work is not going to get you very far. The polarity you are creating in your vibrations is contradicting. Continue your work on gratitude and be consistent on the vibrations of energy you are allowing flow from within you. Only then will you see true transformation from the universe towards your goals and intentions in life.

The Law of Rhythm

Everything has rhythms. The earth and its seasons, the moon and its cycles, your body and mind. Everything has a rhythm that it flows to. The rhythms go up and down, become high and low.

To embrace this law in the best way that you can is to accept you will go through rhythms and cycles many times in life. We like to think we are steady, stable, and maybe even unchanging. That is not reality. Even within our family-ties there are rhythms. Your mannerisms, no doubt, match those of your guardians. Your verbiage of speech are rhythms of the ones you spend the most time around. The cycles of family and the rhythms of speech continue to evolve and change and are rhythmic. To allow yourself to flow alongside the rhythms you naturally are inclined to will bring about a deepening of inner peace.

Think of the ocean. The waves and the stillness that comes in between each wave. When you are swimming in the ocean you come to terms with the waves breaking over your head. And when the waves stop and there is a calmness for a moment, you don't smack the waves and demand more. You have the understanding they will come. When life's rhythm comes, it's best to not force your way through them. You may enjoy being on top of the wave and when the stillness comes it brings about anxiety and fear. Sit with it. Allow yourself to feel the full weight of the stillness within the rhythm you are in and have confidence you will one day be back on top of that wave again.

Take some time to access your inner rhythms. Do you find them to be loud, constant, unstable? Are your inner rhythms more inclined to peace, calm, and understanding? To understand your inner rhythms is to understand yourself better.

The Law of Gender

The Law of Gender extends far past the old social understanding of gender and sex. It has to do with the gender of nature, words, attributes. To say that the world acts in both feminine and masculine ways is to accept the Law of Gender.

Some people have described cultures as either hot or cold. The deeper meaning when someone says this is really that culture depends more on welcoming and hospitality or on productivity and pursuit. The Western culture is mainly described as a cold culture. Of course this depends on which culture you live in and which country you're from. The United States of America is a cold culture. The aim for work, family, and even fun is mainly based on productivity. In contrast, India is a warm culture. If you have ever visited they, culturally, are more concerned about welcoming guests, eating meals with longevity, and not too concerned about time management. These are, of course, stereotypes of the cultures as a whole but one is colder and one is warmer. Another way to say it is one is more masculine and one feminine. Even when depicting texts and poetry in English there are masculine and feminine words and sounds. A ‗g' is considered a harsher letter compared to a ‗p' which is quieter and less abrasive.

This law isn't about what gender someone is or isn't but about the energy that person or yourself is giving off at a given point in time. There really isn't a guide on how to put this law into action in a similar way to the Law of Rhythm, but is more about the intuition this law comes with.

To understand this law is the best course of action to implement it into your life. Once you can identify what is feminine and masculine, you will have an easier time understanding the vibrations you are giving or receiving.

For example, if you have an idea that appears in your head that is feminine. The action you take to put that idea to use is masculine. To explain this further let's talk about decorating a house. You're staring at a blank wall, a canvas, and you have the idea or impression that yellow should be the color of the wall. That is feminine. When you decide to leave the house, drive to the store, and purchase that paint is the masculine action.

When you are flooded with emotions the initial shock of fear, sadness, or joy is a feminine energy. When you decide how to deal with and what to do with those emotions it becomes a masculine energy.

To fully bring the Law of Gender into being within yourself is to recognize the balance of both. To be fully masculine is to be brutish, productive, and faster. To be feminime is to be dainty, fair, and slower. To be fully one or the other is to throw off the balance of life. Everybody has at some level a gist of both genders they hold within themselves but to create autonomy and balance within yourself is to accept that both are needed, necessary, and beautiful.

Summary of How to Integrate the 12 Universal Laws

We just walked through a lot and it can feel overwhelming. The goal of knowing the 12 Universal Laws is not to exercise all of them without fault or constantly be practicing all at once. The goal is to be aware of what you are capable of and bring awareness to your life. Take the concepts of each law and integrate them into your life as it seems fit to yourself. You may want to focus and study one as best you can until you move onto the next. Just remember this is your journey.

We have talked multiple times about meditation and walked through it extensively in the previous chapters. If you have noticed, the practice of meditation can be beneficial on more than just one occasion. You can implement it into steadying your inner being and focusing on gratitude. You can bring about awareness to your own perception of your reality to help you succeed in the practice of the Law of Relativity. Even creating it as a rhythm of your daily activities will help you obtain your goals and self-confidence.

Take a few minutes and read back through each universal law. Is there one besides the Law of Attraction you would like to study more in depth next? Get in tune with who you are and what your intentions are in life. And don't forget to send gratitude out to all that come across your path. You'll be on the road to a fuller and more whole life quicker than you know.

Conclusion

We just went through a lot. Give yourself some gratitude for taking the time, effort, and dedication to improve the quality of your inner and outer being through the Law of Attraction.

When you set a high goal for yourself, you know that it will take a lot of time and dedication to achieve what you have your heart set to. The most important thing for your journey is to have the right tools in your hands. With studying, dedication, and a desire to see your life flourish before your eyes, you will be able to create a new reality you could only dream of for yourself. When dreaming up what you want your life to look like and creating a vision board, don't be afraid to let your heart soar to all the possibilities you can achieve. To create the best outcome for yourself make sure your dreams and goals are precise and well thought out. The universe is intuitive and will know what you are desiring even if you don't. So it's best to get on the same page with what your inner being is desiring and what your outer world is pursuing.

I hope this guide has been as much of a help to you as my own journey through the Law of Attraction has been to me.

Keep in mind that what you give will be what you get in life. To manifest your dreams and desires for your life, focus on the inner work that is needed to achieve those things. I hope you have only felt and received good vibrations of energy through this guide.

References

Bauer, B. (2021, February 17). *Simple practical strategies to feel better now* -. Shambhala Mountain Center. https://blog.shambhalamountain.org/simple-practical-strategies-to-feel-better-now/?gclid=EAIaIQobChMIguHfweCc8gIVNhmtBh3ccAmMEAAYASAAEgL19_D_BwE

Can your diet affect your sleep? (n.d.). Www.piedmont.org. https://www.piedmont.org/living-better/can-your-diet-affect-your-sleep

Coaching. (n.d.). Manifested Harmony. Retrieved August 20, 2021, from https://manifestedharmony.com/law-of-attraction/

EMDR Institute. (2019). *What is EMDR? | EMDR Institute – EYE MOVEMENT DESENSITIZATION AND REPROCESSING THERAPY*. Emdr.com. https://www.emdr.com/what-is-emdr/

Headspace. (2020). *What are all the types of meditation & which one is best?* Headspace. https://www.headspace.com/meditation/techniques

Hurst, K. (2019, June 5). *Law of attraction history: The origins of the law of attraction uncovered*. The Law of Attraction. https://www.thelawofattraction.com/history-law-attraction-uncovered/

Law of Attraction | Harmony | Maria Heals. (2014, June 28). Maria Heals. https://mariaheals.com/law-attraction-harmony/

Law of cause and effect, cosmic law of action, karmic ripples. (n.d.). Open College. Retrieved August 20, 2021, from https://www.opencollege.info/law-of-cause-and-effect/

Life sucks - What are you going to do about it? (n.d.). Www.who-Am-i-Question.com. Retrieved August 20, 2021, from https://www.who-am-i-question.com/life-sucks.html

Smith, A. (2016, November 17). *6 steps to discover your true self*. SUCCESS. https://www.success.com/6-steps-to-discover-your-true-self/

Smith, C. (n.d.). *How to use EFT tapping with the law of attraction – Law of attraction resource guide*. Law of attraction resource guide. Retrieved August 20, 2021, from https://www.lawofattractionresourceguide.com/how-to-use-eft-tapping-with-the-law-of-attraction/

Taylor, A. (2020, August 12). *50 Self-Love journaling prompts for self-discovery & reflection*. Taylor's Tracks. https://www.taylorstracks.com/self-love-journaling-prompts/

Vamos, J. (2019, June 14). *How to manifest love: 7 ways to use the law of attraction to find a relationship*. PairedLife - Relationships. https://pairedlife.com/dating/How-to-Manifest-Love-7-Ways-to-Use-the-Law-of-Attraction-to-Find-a-Relationship

What is access bars? (n.d.). Transformation seeker's guide. Retrieved August 20, 2021, from https://www.practical-personal-development-advice.com/what-is-access-bars.html

Image References

Azevedo, Naasom. (September 25, 2017). *Orando no bosque.* Unsplash. https://unsplash.com/photos/4lrj6z4nRfo

Chaturvedula, Shashi. *Meditation pose.* Unsplash. https://unsplash.com/photos/FjYwhowyp6k

Content Pixie. *A swing in front of a spa in Bali.* Unsplash. https://unsplash.com/photos/2V5PJgGqyts

Deas-Melesh, Taylor. (March 17, 2020). *Young woman doing yoga in a creek in Georgia.* Unsplash. https://unsplash.com/photos/U2EgiLE0ODs

G., Danny (September 11, 2018). *Woman covered in white blankets.* Unsplash. https://unsplash.com/photos/_Utk8ZYT4tI

Hudson, Debby. (December 27, 2018). *Celebrating the sunset.* Unsplash. https://unsplash.com/photos/VIr-KKzL2eg

Janssens, Estée. (September 1, 2018). *Flatlay photography.* Unsplash. https://unsplash.com/photos/MUf7Ly04sOI

Juarez, Lesly. (July 10, 2017). *Mindfulness.* Unsplash. https://unsplash.com/photos/DFtjXYd5Pto

Leon. (May 9, 2019). *Woman in brown long-sleeved.* Unsplash. https://unsplash.com/photos/X8H8vPcelPk

Theodore, Jen. (July 8, 2018). *Black card photo.* Unsplash. https://unsplash.com/photos/hbkWMj41Y0I

www.ingramcontent.com/pod-product-compliance
Lightning Source LLC
Chambersburg PA
CBHW051601010526
44118CB00023B/2780